SMALL STEPS EVERY DAY

The Simple Path To Fitness Success For Busy Adults Over 40

Jack Ward, M.D.

Fitness Publishing

Published by Fitness Marketing Group, Sunrise Beach, MO.

Printed in the United States of America

ISBN: 9781088109656

Disclaimer: The content in this book is for information purposes only and is designed to provide accurate and authoritative information with regard to the subject matter covered. It does not claim to provide medical advice or to be able to treat any medical condition. It makes no claims with respect to any health conditions or to weight loss, either in terms of the amount or rate at which weight loss is achieved. If you have any concerns regarding your health, please contact your medical practitioner before making changes.

First edition

For more information, contact:

Bopp Optimal Health

3421 N. Causeway Blvd. Suite 102

Metairie, LA 70002

1 (318) 550-0050

Visit us online at: **www.PairODocsOnline.com**

Contents

Introduction

THIS BOOK EXISTS FOR two reasons:

Reason #1: So that you'll eventually let me help you implement everything you read here.

Reason #2: To get results in advance so that you'll actually want to do Reason #1 as quickly as possible.

As you'll soon find out, I'm going to be fully transparent, honest, and blunt with you through the pages of this book. My early mentor taught me that if you want people to believe you can help them, help them.

I want to help you.

I'm going to share with you many of the steps and strategies included in my personalized programs for my clients, from top to bottom.

These are the same strategies and methods I personally use to help my clients create the best versions of themselves, while adding very little extra time to their already busy schedules. I'm excited to share it with you here.

It might sound like a lot, but really, the entirety of this book can be summed up in the following three points:

Point #1: It's a busy world and most people don't have (or want to spend) a ton of time to exercise. As they get into the golden years, they want to spend time with their family, enjoying hobbies, traveling the world, or even working more (if that's your thing, no judging).

Point #2: The sooner you incorporate a health and nutrition program seamlessly into your life, the sooner your quality of life improves, allowing you to live your life as the very best version of you... regardless of age.

Point #3: The best method to effortlessly integrate a simple, timesaving, results-proven approach to increasing the longevity and quality of your life is the one you'll find in this very book. I call it **Small Steps Every Day**.

The methods and strategies you're about to discover has radically transformed my life for the better, with benefits far beyond health and fitness. I hope you'll be able to make the connection for yourself as well. Above all, it is my sincere hope that you learn more than just how to implement the strategies and tactics in **Small Steps Every Day**.

I've interspersed little bits of advice and lessons I've learned from over thirty years on the front lines of the fitness industry, having made all the mistakes and living to tell the tale.

Yes, this is a health and nutrition book, but it's really a book about designing a better life. A life that brings you joy, financial rewards, and even peace.

I sincerely believe that the world can, should, and will be changed for the better within my lifetime and the lifetime of my family. I believe it will be the entrepreneurs, self-employed, dreamers, and innovators like you who will make that happen.

So, it's a great privilege to share what I know with you. I hope it inspires and informs you to grow and improve your own life, so you can grow and improve the lives of others.

It is my sincere hope that by teaching you the **Small Steps Every Day** principles, you will be able to develop a better version of you that delivers exactly what you need in your life to lift, inspire, and serve others. In return, you will live a higher quality of life than you could ever imagine, even during difficult times. Because when times get hard, people need even more help than usual. By following the methods in this book, you'll discover a sure-fire method to get twice the results in half the time.

And of course, above all else, it is my sincere hope that by taking the time to read this short book, you will see a path forward to not only better health and fitness achievement but also for more peace. After all, what's the point in being healthy if you can't enjoy life with the ones you love in the way you want.

So, my friend, this book is for everyone approaching or in their golden years who wants live their best life but are ready to do it the right way through a simple and strategic program, rather than accepting the aging process and enduring a lifestyle far below what they deserve.

If you read this book and decide you'd like help implementing its strategies as quickly as possible, please feel free to call and chat with me and my team by going here:

(318) 550-0050

Helping people like you to create the highest and best version of themselves is exactly what I do day-in and day-out.

I'm here to help.

To your success,

Jack Ward, M.D.

Chapter 1

Your Attitude Determines Your Altitude

S UCCESS IN ANY EXERCISE program... *and in LIFE, for that matter*... depends largely on the attitude that a person brings to his endeavors. I want to touch on the importance of a positive mindset in achieving your ideal body.

That's because it all starts in your head. Every day, we make hundreds of choices, starting with whether to get out of bed or not. Some choices contribute to achieving our dreams, and others keep us away from them. And even when we **DON'T** make a choice, we already have... by choosing not to. *Our choices, and the actions that follow, add up to make us the people we are.* In fact, we are the total of all the choices that we have made during our lives, right up to this very moment.

I believe that like a muscle, the mind can be trained. Motivation to accomplish all of your goals can be built just like a muscle, a little at a time. The more you work on building your motivation and developing a positive mindset, the stronger you become as a person.

I'll give you an example. Whenever I travel on an airplane, I seldom take the time to talk to the person next to me. But I'll never forget this one man that sat next to me. He looked terribly down, so I asked him, *"How are you?"* He said, *"Oh, okay, I guess."* Then he asked me, *"What do you do for a living?"*

I said I was a personal trainer, but some people might call me a motivational speaker since that is a lot of what my job entails. I motivate people to be their physical best. Then, right out of nowhere, he asked,

"Tell me something. **Why does everything go wrong for me?"**

Well, I certainly didn't know. I had never met the man before. So I replied,

"Beats me."

For the next thirty minutes, he went on and on about all his difficulties. There I was, stuck on a crowded airplane, listening to this man I've never seen before. And he repeated the same negative thoughts over and over again.

Then suddenly he exclaimed,

*"Hold it! Hold it! I know why everything goes wrong for me. It just came to me. **Everything goes wrong for me because I'm wrong.** I think wrong, speak wrong, and act wrong. I'm just too negative all the time."*

He was right. He had gotten right to the crux of the matter.

It was his attitude that was determining his altitude.

The same is true for you. Your attitude is one of the most important, most powerful factors in your life. In fact, just about everything you achieve or don't achieve can be traced back to your attitude. Quite simply, good attitudes bring good results, and bad attitudes bring bad results. **It is your attitude, more than your aptitude that will determine your altitude.**

YOU ARE WHAT YOU THINK!

Of course, a lot of people think it's "cool" to joke about one's attitude.

Comedian George Burns was once asked,

"Can you do everything at 98 you could do at age 18?"

He said,

"Of course I can do everything at 98 I did at 18 - which tells you how pathetic my life was at 18."

Sure, it can be fun to joke about a negative attitude, but in reality, nothing could be more serious.

Benjamin Franklin knew that. He said,

"Most people die at age 18, but we don't bury them until they're 65."

Think about that!

It's like a point that a psychologist made to me a few years ago. He asked me,

"How long have you been alive?"

I responded something like,

"43 years."

Then he said,

*"No. That's how long your heart has been beating. How long have you been **ALIVE**? How long have you been on fire?"*

About that time I "got" it. The light bulb came on. I realized what he was getting at.

It's a person's attitude that pushes them forward or holds them back.

Of course, you may be thinking that all this talk about attitude is just a bunch of pie-in-the-sky talk. Is there any evidence to back up my claims? Yup. ***Absolutely!***

In one long-term study of 1500 people, group A - or 83%-- of the people took their particular jobs because they believed they could make lots of money. Only 17% of them - or group B - took their particular jobs because they happened to have a positive attitude towards those jobs.

Twenty years later, the two groups had produced 101 millionaires. The amazing thing is, only one of those millionaires came from group A, but 100 of them came from group B.

Now that's significant!

Even more amazing, over 70% of these millionaires never went to college. And over 70% of those who became CEOs graduated in the bottom half of their class. The conclusion was that it was their attitude, more than their aptitude, that determined their altitude. ***In no uncertain terms***, this study determined that positive thinking is "the" hallmark of successful people.

My psychologist friend from above made this point even clearer to me. He explained that he asks clients to give him the words they would use to characterize a winner, and then he'll write down the first ten words they give him.

What do you think they say?

Over the years, he found their answers to be very consistent. They list:

- attitude,

- enthusiasm,

- determination,

- motivation,

- confidence,

- optimism,

- dedication,

- happiness,

- balance,

- and patience.

Very interesting.

None of these qualities has anything to do with physical or mental abilities. They all relate to attitude in some way or another.

You're obviously interested in physical fitness. You want to build the best body possible. Well, your attitude has a lot to do with your physical success as well.

Most people think of mind and body as two separate realms when, in effect, they are part of the same whole. In order to have a healthy body, you must have a healthy mind. ***Sometimes the best medicine is in your head.***

One of the first people to popularize the mind-body connection was Norman Cousins. As a respected journalist and professor, he wrote and spoke on the topic many times. One study was particularly interesting, a study done on 40 patients who recovered from "irreversible" illnesses.

When they were told they had little a chance to live, they panicked. That was to be expected.

Recent battles with health problems had me fully understanding the emotions and feeling of despair that come with such a diagnosis. I found myself making plans for the inevitable during that recent period. Life insurance, trusts, wills, etc. These things become matters that consume one's mind when they prepare for the "inevitable."

But at some point, those 40 patients decided to reject the notion of foreseeable death. ***They decided to live!*** They would take advantage of the best that medical science had to offer, but they would also get actively involved in their own recovery. They would do whatever it took to regain their health.

According to Cousins, it was that decision, ***that attitude***, which made the difference. Attitudes have a definite biochemical effect on the body. An attitude of defeat or panic constricts the blood vessels and has a debilitating effect on the entire endocrine system. By contrast, an attitude of confidence and determination activates benevolent, therapeutic secretions in the brain.

Apparently, a positive attitude can help in the prevention of disease, and a positive attitude can help in the recovery from disease. Dr. James Strain, the director of Behavioral Medicine and Consultation Psychiatry at Mount Sinai Hospital in New York City, found that to be true. Dr. Strain compared pessimistic and optimistic men who had heart attacks. In the first group of 25, 21 of the 25 pessimistic men died within 8 years of their heart attack. But only 6 of the 25 optimistic men died during that time.

Yes, I'm a physician. But you don't have to be a doctor to see a definite connection between the mind and body. It's pretty obvious to me that when faced with an "inevitable," when the facts won't budge, you have to change your attitude. You may have no power to change the "facts" in your world, but you **_always_** have the power to change your response to those "facts," and that power can be enormous.

More often than not, your attitude is the number one determining factor in your success. With the right attitude, you're almost certain to achieve your goals. And the good news is, **_your attitude is self- chosen_**. You control whether you will be a winner in life, or not, regardless of your natural ability.

So you can be a winner. You can have a stronger body. You can have better relationships. You can make more money—if you have the right attitude. **_It is your responsibility to change your attitude_** if it's not as positive or as powerful as it needs to be. No one "gave" you your attitude, and no one can "take" it away—except you.

It's your responsibility.

I'm sure you want to be a "winner." You don't want to be a "loser." ***And the difference between the two is huge.***

The winner is always a part of the answer.

The loser is always a part of the problem.

The winner always has a program.

The loser always has an excuse.

The winner says, "Let me help you."

The loser says, "That's not my job."

The winner sees an answer for every problem.

The loser sees a problem in every answer.

The winner sees a green near every sand trap.

The loser sees a sand trap near every green.

The winner says, "It may be difficult, but it's possible."

The loser says, "It may be possible, but it's too difficult."

Can you think of a bigger winner than Abraham Lincoln? I can't think of anyone who had more pressures in life or in his career than Abraham Lincoln. Whether it was his repeated losses in various elections, his difficult marriage, or the nation falling apart, he lived and led with an indomitable positive attitude.

He simply chose to be that way.

As Lincoln said,

"Most people are about as happy as they make up their minds to be."

Starting today, I'm making up my mind to be like Abe! How about you?

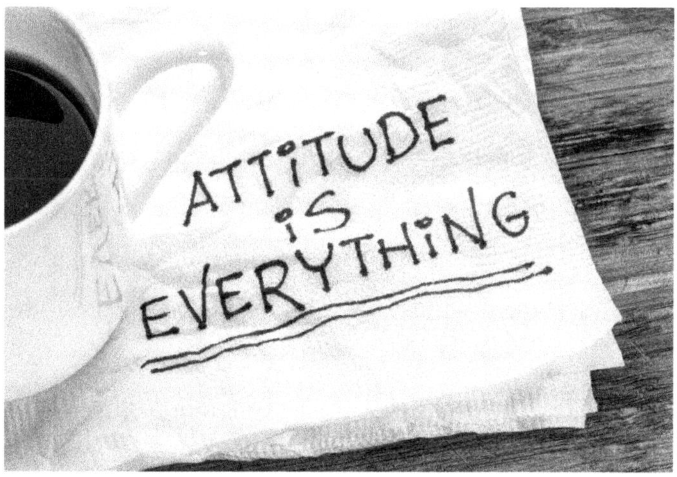

Chapter 2

Quick Fix, Fast Failure

WE LIVE IN A quick-fix society. When we want something, we want it now!

Worse, we're constantly presented with ways to lose weight immediately — advertisements convince us that we can lose inches by tomorrow, and be slimmer by next week. There's no harm in wanting to lose weight by yesterday. After all, it's possible, isn't it?

NO! Not at all. When it comes down to it, fast weight loss cannot last, because it usually means adapting to very difficult eating habits and an impossible-to-live with lifestyle. Plus, with quick-fix diets, our metabolism slows down, and eventually we're eating fewer and fewer calories but not losing weight. This leads to anxiety, which prompts us to eat even fewer calories to try losing the weight. The body rebels against that even more.

So it becomes a vicious cycle. Because if you don't get enough nutrients — which is a major risk when you're going for a quick fix — your brain, and then your body, will, well, insist that you eat. To your body, it's nothing more than survival. But to you, it will feel like you're giving into cravings and losing control. Then you'll feel shame and failure, which might very well send you to the fridge.

It's a never-ending Yo-Yo cycle of weight gain, then weight loss, then weight gain again.

If we strive for slow and steady weight loss, on the other hand (a healthy rate of weight loss is two pounds per week or less), not only will you be doing a service to your body, you'll be more likely to keep that weight off for good. Isn't that better than rebounding?

Chapter 3

Why Slow Weight Loss Lasts

IT'S THAT KIND OF "through thick and thin" attitude that will take people from thick to thin for good. Losing weight slowly isn't just healthier, it's a better investment. Not only are you shedding pounds, you're working on building habits you'll be able to maintain. And those habits will help you maintain the weight you lost, so you can stay at your weight goal for good.

Plus, you will have more energy to live life in the present, because you're not starving and focusing on food. You're creating a healthy relationship with food, so food will become your friend rather than your enemy. That's the key to lifelong success.

Additionally, we know to distance ourselves from the standards set by super-models, actors, and actresses. We remind ourselves that they employ stylists, makeup artists, gourmet chefs specializing in low-fat cooking, and personal trainers to keep them toned and lean.

However, it's not so easy to abandon those negative thoughts and comparisons when the picture of progress and health is sitting right next to us on the couch. There are times when it seems as if everyone in our healthy-lifestyle circle is dropping pounds or knocking back dress sizes while, despite our best broiled-chicken efforts, we remain unchanged.

But don't let this heart-breaker defeat your good intentions. With the right mental attitude, you can use this experience to bolster your own progress.

We are all different in every way, and that's especially true with weight loss. Weight loss isn't neat and tidy. It comes in spurts. Over time, it's significant, and you need to establish your own winning goal and focus on that. Don't compare yourself with others.

Remembering that we all lose weight at our own rate provides an opportunity to learn about the beauty of individuality. The most devastating thing we can do when setting a goal for weight loss is to compare our success or progress to others. We are all individuals, not clones who respond like Pavlov dogs or mice, to the same experiment.

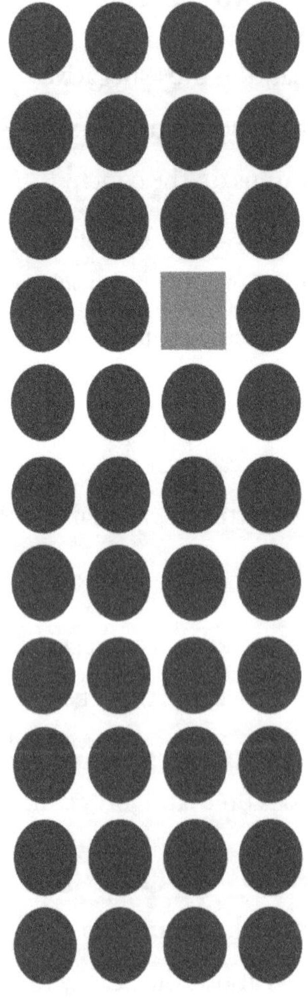

Not going along with the crowd can help you stand out in the crowd.

Sometimes being yourself is the hardest thing to do. Going along with the crowd may be easy, but being an individual is more rewarding. Don't make your choices based on the crowd. Make your choices based on *your* feelings... *your* values... and *your* needs!

Chapter 4

Our Bodies, Our Weight Loss

IT'S ALSO IMPORTANT TO remember that it's never the same experiment. Dieting history, medications, age, activity level, our percentage of lean body mass, and stress level all play roles in a person's weight loss. In other words, your weight loss will differ from everyone else's.

Additionally, in the first few weeks of any weight-loss program, losses typically are greater because of lost water weight. **The important thing to remember is that the overall average should be somewhere between one-half to two pounds a week.**

Envision yourself a year from today wearing the clothes you want to wear. A pound a week in a year is 52 pounds. *That's impressive!*

Finally, you didn't gain weight overnight, so don't expect to lose weight overnight, either. Be patient. The payoff will be well worth the wait.

The number of people in the United States who are overweight has increased over the last two decades. **Current estimates are that over seventy percent of adults and forty percent of children and teenagers in the United States are overweight.** Obesity is a primary causal factor in a wide range of serious diseases, including heart disease, stroke, and some types of cancer. It also tends to raise your blood pressure and cholesterol levels, and makes you more likely to develop diabetes. Hence, obesity is one of the most significant *and preventable* causes of death and disability among adults.

The number of calories you eat and the number of calories you burn each day control your body weight. **It is that simple!**

Calories in vs. Calories out.

So to lose weight, you need to take in fewer calories than you burn. You can do this by becoming more physically active, by eating less or a combination of both. Your weight loss program should also help you make changes you can maintain for the rest of your life. **Diets don't work...** *lifestyle changes work!!!*

LOST:

SMALL WHITE POODLE Last seen on East Main Street. Reward! Please call 555-1212

WANTED:

SOMEONE TO LOVE ME FOR ME. Looking for a person who can understand me like no one else can. Someone who will appreciate my uniqueness and respect my opinions. Love and understanding are a must. Wanting to develop a life-long relationship.

FOUND:

LARGE BROWN COLLIE Found

If you're looking for someone to love, start by looking in the mirror!

Chapter 5

Are You Overweight?

T HE MOST COMMON WAY to decide if you are overweight is to determine your Body Mass Index (BMI). The BMI looks at how much you should weigh based on your height. It is a relative comparison of the proportion of fat versus lean muscle on your body.

> **You can determine your BMI by using the following formula:**
>
> 1. Divide your weight (in pounds) by your height (in inches) squared.
> 2. Multiply the result of Step 1 by 705.
>
> For example, if you are 5'3" (63 inches) and weigh 138 pounds, the equation looks like this:
>
> $$BMI = [138/(63 \times 63)] \times 705 = 24.5$$

Your BMI should be somewhere in the 19 to 25 range. A BMI of 25 to 29.9 is considered overweight and a BMI of over 30 is considered obese. If you are not sure whether you are overweight, see your doctor.

If you decide you need to lose weight, where should you start? **First and foremost, you should concentrate on eating a healthy diet.** Consider what you are eating. ***Unequivocally, nutrition is 70%-80% of the equation necessary to lose body fat.*** To lose weight while remaining healthy, you should try to lose only about 1/2 to 2 pounds per week. **One pound equals 3,500 calories.** So if you cut out or exercise off 500 calories per day, you will lose about a pound a week. Losing weight will be easier if you combine exercise with diet management and good nutrition.

Nutrition

A good diet has a structure known as the food pyramid. The idea behind the food pyramid is not necessarily to exclude any particular food, but to eat more of the healthy foods, and less of the unhealthy, fattening foods. You should eat more of the foods at the bottom, largest layer of the pyramid.

- **Grain Group** - breads, cereals, rices, pastas and other foods made from grain. They provide B vitamins, iron, carbohydrates and some proteins.

- **Fruit and Vegetable Group** - Most vitamins, minerals, and fiber can be found in this group.

- **Dairy and Meat Group** - This group contains foods with a lot of protein. Some foods are milk, cheese, poultry, fish and eggs, as well as nuts and beans. In addition to protein, these foods have calcium, iron, phosphorus, B vitamins and zinc.

- **Fats, Oils and Sweets Group** - The foods in this group provide calories, but little nutritional benefit. They include salad dressing, butter, margarine, sugar, sodas and candy. The American Heart Association recommends that no more than 30% of calories come from fats per day.

The American Dietetic Association lists several warning signs to look for in a diet that signals bad nutritional advice:

- Recommendations that promise a quick fix

- Dire warnings of dangers from a single product or regimen

- Claims that sound too good to be true

- Simplistic conclusions drawn from a complex study

- Recommendations based on a single study

- Dramatic statements that are refuted by reputable scientific organizations

- Lists of "good" and "bad" foods

- Recommendations made to help sell a product

- Recommendations based on studies published without peer review

- Recommendations from studies that ignore differences among individuals or groups

Variety is the spice of life! Eating a variety of foods helps provide vitamins, minerals and fiber, all of which may help reduce chronic disease risk. ***You don't need to give up favorite foods when trying to maintain or lose weight***, but you may need to eat less of it less often. Some tips on eating well and losing weight:

- Choose low fat, low-calorie foods. Eat grilled fish instead of fried fish; instead of french fries, have a baked potato (without all the butter and sour cream).

- Try to limit your serving size and actually measure out the portions of food you are going to eat. It is very easy to overestimate how much you are eating. Keep measuring cups and spoons at the ready.

- Eat a variety of foods for maximum nutritional benefit.

- If you want to be able to eat more food while losing weight, the answer is **EXERCISE**.

Recommended Foods For Weight-Loss Success

PROTEIN	COMPLEX CARBOHYDRATES	FIBROUS CARBOHYDRATES
chicken breast	baked potato	broccoli
turkey breast	sweet potato	cauliflower
lean ground turkey	yam	asparagus
top round steak	steamed brown rice	lettuce
top sirloin steak	steamed wild rice	carrots
lean ground beef	steamed white rice	green beans
swordfish	oatmeal	green peppers
egg whites or substitute	pasta	mushrooms
orange roughy	beans	spinach
tuna	corn	onions
salmon	strawberries	peas
crab	melon	celery
lobster	apple	cabbage
shrimp	orange	zucchini
low-fat cottage cheese	fat-free yogurt	artichoke
	whole wheat bread	

Choose a portion of protein and complex carbohydrates from each column to make a meal. Add a serving of fibrous carbohydrates to at least two of your daily meals.

9 RULES FOR SUCCESSFUL WEIGHT LOSS

- Eat 4-6 small meals per day, preferably every 2-3 hours.

- Eat one portion of protein and complex carbohydrates with every meal.

- Add fibrous carbohydrates to at least 2 meals.

- A portion of food is approximately the size of your palm or clenched fist.

- Drink at least 8 glasses of water each day.

- Use Meal Replacement Shakes whenever necessary to ensure you are consuming the optimal levels of required nutrients.

- Plan your meals in advance and record what you eat.

- Plan your grocery list.

- Once a week give yourself a free day to eat _whatever_ you want.

Exercise

Regular physical activity will not only help you lose weight, but you will look and feel better. Exercise will lower your blood pressure and cholesterol, it can reduce your risk of having a heart attack and will temporarily suppress your appetite! **Any activity that is done for at least 30 minutes on most days will help**. You should try to exercise aerobically, meaning hard enough to make your heart pound a little and make you breathe heavier. If you are so out of breath that you can't comfortably talk to someone, you are exercising too hard. **Slow down!** To burn the maximum amount of fat, you should exercise at a lower intensity for a longer period.

FACT AND FICTION ABOUT DIET & EXERCISE

FACT: To transform you physique you <u>must</u> train with weights.
FICTION: Aerobics is better for shaping up than weights.

If you don't train with weights your skin will have nothing to "shape" around when the aerobics and diet program reduces body fat.

FACT: If you exercise, it matters even more what you eat.
FICTION: If you exercise, it doesn't matter what you eat.

When you exercise your body requires more calories to compensate for the energy expended.

FACT: Weight training helps women "tone up," creating lean bodies.
FICTION: If women lift weights, they will get "bulky."

Women do not produce enough testosterone to get big, bulky muscles.

FACT: People of all ages should be weight training.
FICTION: Weight training is only for younger people.

Studies show that older people benefit _even more_ from weight training than younger people.

FACT: Muscles grow while you are resting and recuperating.
FICTION: Muscles grow while you are working out.

Working out actually tears down muscles. They grow, or "shape," while they are resting.

FACT: Your body _always_ needs more water than it is telling you.
FICTION: You need to drink water only when you are thirsty.

If you are thirsty, your body is already in a dehydrated state.

FACT: There is no such thing as eating "perfectly."
FICTION: You have to eat perfectly all the time.

FACT: Studies do show that many of us need to take supplements.
FICTION: If you eat right you do not need to take supplements.

Most people are lacking in some vitamins and nutrients from their personal food consumption.

Summary

Exercise and eating well, when combined, are the most effective means of losing and maintaining weight. **Period!** To get you on your way to losing weight, try using these strategies:

- Monitor your weight and food intake. Depending on your personality, you may prefer to weigh yourself every week as opposed to every day. Use measuring cups to measure out food portions since it is very easy to overestimate amounts of food.

- Plan your meals ahead of time and have small, healthy snacks if necessary so that you don't become so hungry that you overeat. **A healthy snack is something like a piece of fruit or a handful of raisins or nuts.**

- Try to focus on your internal hunger signals instead of external stimuli telling you to eat. Don't eat if you are not hungry, even if that is the time you normally would eat. You can resist cravings for foods in between meals by doing something to take your mind off eating.

Try taking a walk or doing something active to distract yourself until the craving passes.

- Try to avoid high-risk situations where you would tend to overeat. When you feel tired, lonely, bored, depressed, or anxious, you are more likely to eat when you are not hungry.

- Try waiting 10 minutes if you have eaten your meal and you are still hungry. Give your meal time to "catch up with you." Cravings for snacks may also pass if you tell yourself to wait 10 minutes or so before you give in.

Losing weight can be very hard, and it can take time. **Just remember that you didn't gain weight overnight, and you won't lose it overnight either.** If, after several months of eating right and exercising, you still are not losing weight, you may decide to see your doctor. Most people are capable of losing weight on their own, without medical intervention.

REMEMBER: *Almost anyone can lose weight!!!* Weight loss is based on the Law of Thermodynamics which simply translated refers to the relationship of calories in vs. Calories out... if you burn more calories than you eat, you **WILL LOSE WEIGHT**... if you eat more calories than you burn, you **WILL GAIN WEIGHT**. It's really that simple.

The aim is to allow you to eat as much as possible, and move as little as possible to allow you to reach your personal weight-loss goal. **That is perfect!!!**

Chapter 6

Sample Diet Program

SAMPLE DIET PROGRAM

8:00 AM	Breakfast	2 oz. Oatmeal 16 oz. water Apple (optional)
10:00 AM	Mid-morning	Banana, Protein Drink or Protein Bar
1:00 PM	Lunch	4-6 oz. of lean meat (Chicken, turkey, fish, lean beef) 4 oz. vegetable 16 oz. water
4:00 PM	Mid-afternoon	Apple, Protein Drink or Protein Bar
6:00 PM	Dinner	4-6 oz. of lean meat (Chicken, turkey, fish, lean beef) 16 oz. water
8:00 PM	Evening	4-6 oz. lean meat (Chicken, turkey, fish, lean beef) Small salad 16 oz. water

Chapter 7

Eight Ways To Avoid Cheating On A Diet

W E'VE ALL DONE IT. Sneaked an extra piece of cake when nobody was looking. Nobody, that is, except the cat. And who was he going to tell? Or we might say that we're running out of the office for a minute to pick up something from the drugstore, or the newspaper stand, or the ... Oh! Heck, what does it matter? And instead we go to the new candy shop down the street.

Some call it "cheating." Some call it "sneaking." Others call it "closet eating." But one of the reasons dieters "cheat" is that they're often so strict with themselves that they end up feeling deprived.

Remember that healthy eating includes lots of "good" choices with a few "naughty" ones as well. Devising some strategies to help you enjoy treats rather than "cheat" will help keep you on the straight and narrow path. Here are some suggestions:

Plan for treats. Making sure you enjoy your favorite treats every once in a while will help you from feeling deprived. Pick a night each week, **ONLY ONE NIGHT,** when you can indulge in something decadent like a piece of chocolate mud cake. ***Give yourself permission to truly enjoy your dessert!*** Taking the time to savor a treat is always more satisfying than gobbling it down with feelings of guilt or shame.

Put your food cupboard on a diet. If most of the foods that enter your house are healthy, then the battle is almost won. If you must have tempting foods around for a special occasion, store them out of sight or buy them at the last minute. On the big day, enjoy your favorite foods and send any leftovers home with your guests.

Choose your friends wisely. Beware of any "friend" who continually tries to coerce you into *"just a cappuccino"* – which you know really means a cappuccino and a slice of cake with frosting an inch thick. Put those friends on hold until you feel you are strong enough to say "no." Or suggest a different kind of get-together, such as a walk in the park.

Count the cost, as well as the calories. Allocate so many dollars per pound you plan to lose and save the money in a separate account or piggy bank. Or "pay" yourself so much every day that you stick to your weight-loss plan. Then treat yourself to something fabulous, like a new outfit or a day at a beauty spa.

Picture yourself. Find some not-so-flattering photos of yourself and place them strategically at prime temptation spots - the fridge, the cookie jar, or in your desk drawer. That way, you will be reminded of the positive changes you're trying to make to your life whenever you're tempted to over-indulge.

Surround yourself with witnesses. Tell everyone you are changing your eating habits. Give them permission to remind you of your dedication to better health if they catch you transgressing. Beg them to stay on you about it. Make sure you have chosen friends who will support and encourage you. The last thing you need is someone who will try to sabotage your goals. **See #3 above**.

Check up on yourself. Keep a food journal where you write down every single thing that passes through your lips each day. If you often eat when you're upset or stressed, try to record that, too. If you gobbled up a candy bar after arguing with your partner, you probably need to find alternative ways of coping with your moods. Next time try phoning a friend or going for a stress-relieving walk.

Keep a sense of proportion. We all slip up from time to time. We all forget our best resolutions and bend the rules. It's not the end of the world. The worst thing you can do is give in and say, *"Well, I blew it. Let's forget it. I'm never going to succeed."* Now, that would really be cheating. Not just cheating on your diet, but cheating on yourself and your health as well. Just get right back on track. Forget it. Move on.

Chapter 8

The Top Six Weight Loss Lies

WHAT LIES ARE YOU telling yourself as you journey along the road to weight loss? Maybe more than you realize. It's time to get honest, because those untruths may stand in the way of you reaching your aims.

Most people set unrealistic goals or deprive themselves in extreme ways that are very difficult, if not impossible, to maintain. It's no wonder so many people lose weight initially, but then have difficulty keeping the weight off.

Here, we address the most common myths that undermine a healthy approach to weight loss — along with tips on overcoming them to achieve success.

1. **I need to go on a "diet."** The whole concept of a "diet" sets us up to think we will be "on a diet" then "off a diet." Instead, think of your weight-loss plan as a lifestyle commitment to

healthy eating and exercise for the long haul.

2. **I'll get back on track on Monday/after the holidays/whcn the sun comes out.** There's no day like today. If you slip, just pick up where you left off. Persistence works wonders.

3. **All my problems will be solved when I lose weight.** Dropping pounds may leave you feeling healthier and happier — but it won't make you more lovable or turn you into a runway model. **Be clear about why you want to lose weight and set realistic goals.** It's far more motivating to strive toward being fit and energetic than it is to strive toward being a size 2.

4. **Fat people don't deserve to eat.** Do you forego the office pizza because you're afraid people will think you shouldn't be eating? Seeing yourself through others' eyes in a harsh, critical way is a guaranteed way to blow a weight-loss plan. Instead, it's more effective to focus on developing a more loving relationship with your body. A study published in the Journal of Behavioral Medicine (Winter 1998) found that those who started out accepting their bodies were more than

twice as likely to lose weight as those who felt dissatisfied or ashamed.

5. **I shouldn't wear a bathing suit (shorts, a tank top) until I've lost all the weight.** Lots of people of all different sizes enjoy sexy clothes. When you love yourself, you start enjoying life. Break big goals into smaller ones, and reward yourself along the way. Instead of saying, *"I need to lose 25 pounds,"* say, *"I'll buy a new swimsuit when I'm one size smaller."*

6. **The less I eat, the faster I'll lose. *Wrong!*** The less you eat, the slower your metabolism gets, and the slower you will lose the weight. Deprivation also makes us unhappy and actually causes us to overeat and overindulge. A slow and steady approach — including treating yourself to your favorite foods, in moderation — is your best chance for reaching your long-term weight-loss goals.

So stop telling yourself lies that sabotage your efforts. Instead, start living your life with a weight loss plan that works for you. You'll feel better about yourself, your confidence will grow, and you'll keep the weight off.

Procrastination is suicide on the...

Installment Plan!

Most people give up just when they're about to achieve success.

Chapter 9

Six Keys To Fitness Success

T HE FIRST THING I can tell you is that the information in this book will work for you! **I guarantee it!** The exercise information is based on solid research and principles of exercise physiology, and the fat loss information differs greatly from popular weight-loss fads that can be restrictive, unbalanced, and can even set you up for failure after some initial success.

If the prospect of changing your body seems daunting, I'll tell you a secret that's been the basis of every worthwhile goal I've ever reached. The key to success, in anything, isn't extraordinary, superhuman effort. ***It's daily action.*** You find a set of actions that you believe will produce good results if you follow them consistently, and then you follow them consistently. You don't reach a goal by constantly saying, so little done, so much more to do. Just focus on taking small consistent steps, and suddenly you'll discover that you've arrived. The focus should be squarely on the present - "What are the actions I can take today that will bring success?"

You can do this. As you'll see, a good fitness program isn't accidental. All the pieces are explained in this manual, in exact detail. They're specific, and they're crucial. In my view, the following six elements, with no pieces missing, are essential to fast fitness:

1. Cardiovascular exercise (2-4 x weekly, 30-45 minutes per session) - Interval training

2. Resistance training (2-5 x weekly, 25-45 minutes per session)

3. Water!

4. Four to six limited, balanced meals each day

5. Focus on creating a deficit

6. Sufficient rest

Now let me explain these briefly, and in more detail later. If your current program is not working for you, for any reason, you need to add the missing pieces of the puzzle to make it work. **Period!**

Now, before you start feeling overwhelmed, let me assure you that there are appropriate ways to include all of these in your program, regardless of your age, gender or level of fitness. ***The key is starting at the proper level.*** If you're new to exercise, I strongly recommend that you have a conversation with your doctor first, and it's perfectly OK to start slowly.

Let's go through each of the components individually. On the exercise front, the most effective way to get fit is to include a specific variety of exercises in your program. This includes cardiovascular exercise, interval training and resistance training.

THE BEST EXERCISE IS THE ONE YOU....

ACTUALLY DO!

1. Cardiovascular Exercise

Breathe. If you want to measure how many calories someone is burning, with great accuracy, you measure their breathing. One of the first things you can do to improve your health, both physically and mentally, is to become aware of your breathing - both in and out. When you follow your breath, your mind stops running around. If you combine that with awareness of what you're doing - lifting a barbell, playing with your kids, sitting in traffic - you'll experience life in everyday things.

Cardiovascular activity is anything that elevates your oxygen intake, preferably in full, regular breaths. This includes walking, jogging, running, biking, and other activities. By the way, *you'll __always__ get more power if you focus on your breathing and let your speed catch up than if you focus on your speed and let your breathing catch up.*

Here's why you need cardiovascular exercise. Exercise has two functions: one is to trigger metabolic adaptation, and the other is to do mechanical work. Both expend a lot of energy, and if you want to burn a lot of fat, you will want to take advantage of both. The short-duration, high-intensity stuff triggers adaptation (muscle gain, enzyme changes, cellular reorganization, lactate tolerance, cardiovascular improvement). You burn fat afterward in order to replace muscle glycogen. The longer duration, lower intensity aerobic activity (breathing deeply but still "conversational") allows you to create an energy demand that burns fat right then and there. If you include both types, you're going to lose fat fast.

Which exercise is best? Generally, those that engage the largest amount of muscle, including the full lower body. The more muscle groups you engage, the more work your body does, but the less exertion you feel because no single muscle group bears the whole burden. Some of the better choices include walking at a high incline, running (outdoor or treadmill), ski machines, elliptical machines, and stationary bikes that work both arms and legs. Start slow if you're out of shape. Even walking is fine if it elevates your breathing and you focus on using your muscles. Exercises that isolate the arms (like swimming) aren't as effective, but you can also improve those by emphasizing the leg muscles more. Probably the best advice is to pick the exercises you're actually willing to include as part of your lifestyle.

Interval Training

A few times in each cardiovascular workout, you should raise your activity enough to get winded and recover, get winded, and recover again. This is called "interval training." **If you're starting from a very low level of fitness, ease into this!** The goal is progress, not injury. If you're extremely out of shape, a "wind sprint" for you may initially be simply walking up a hill. Be patient - your conditioning will improve. Of course, if just thinking about getting up off the couch is your wind sprint, we've got some work to do. In any case, remember - no gasping allowed.

Scientists measure fitness by a calculation referred to as VO2Max. This is the maximum speed that the body can absorb oxygen. Typically, the faster you recover normal breathing after getting "winded", the more fit you are. So how do you train VO2Max? You do cardiovascular exercise that incorporates periods of activity high enough to get you winded (never gasping), followed by a return to moderate (not low or zero) levels of activity until you recover your regular breathing. These "wind sprints" can be 5 minutes, 1 minute, or even 20 seconds.

2. Resistance Training

Want to raise your metabolism? Start by understanding that aside from a moderate amount of calories burned in digestion, **the main tissue that burns energy in the body is muscle...** ***even at rest!*** The quickest way to lower your metabolism is to lose muscle. **The best and fastest way to raise your metabolism is to build and/or preserve muscle.** Again, done at the proper level, virtually anybody can benefit from including resistance training as part of their fitness program.

Muscle growth is essentially a repair process. The goal in resistance training is not to push a lot of poundage - it's to stress the muscle with very focused contraction (in the concentric or "lifting" phase) and tension (in the eccentric or "lowering" phase) in order to cause micro-tears to the muscles that result in new growth. In order for muscle growth to occur, you have to follow up your training with proper nutrition and rest.

So resistance training, or "bodybuilding" is not just "weight lifting." There's a huge difference between bodybuilding and simply lifting weights. Weight lifting means lifting weights - moving poundage for the sake of moving poundage. Bodybuilding, or resistance training, means more than that. It means being aware of the specific muscle being trained by every exercise, using proper form (especially during the final repetitions when good form is easily lost), focusing on contracting the muscle during the concentric (lifting) movement and creating tension by going slow - at least 2 seconds - during the eccentric (lowering) movement. I don't care how many pounds you can lift if you're swinging the weight without causing contraction and tension in the right muscles.

Here's why you need resistance training. Much less than half of your "fat free mass" (scale weight minus body fat) is active, or skeletal muscle. But that muscle accounts for most of the energy you use daily. A pound of pure muscle burns approximately 50 calories a day (though less at sedentary activity levels). To put that in perspective, a pound of fat is 3500 calories. The more lean muscle you have, the easier it is to burn fat. Suppose somebody goes on a restrictive or unbalanced fad diet, such as Atkins, does nothing to preserve muscle tissue, and loses 10 pounds of muscle (which is not unusual), some fat, and a lot of water. They may look at the scale and think that's progress. But as soon as they go off the diet, the water will rapidly return and the scale weight will shoot back up. Worse, they'll find that a caloric intake that used to keep their weight constant may now cause them to gain as much as a pound of fat a week. ***The less muscle mass you have, the harder it is to lose weight and keep it off!*** So even if your goal is purely fat loss, you've got to keep up the resistance training so that your lean mass at least stays constant.

If you're trying to gain muscle, the intensity of muscle contraction is much more important than duration, and anything more than an hour of intensity will exhaust your glycogen and creatine phosphate stores, which you'll experience as muscle fatigue. ***If you're spending more than an hour training with weights, it's called aerobics!*** You should take only about a minute of rest between sets of the same exercise, and only 2-3 minutes of rest between exercises.

As for safety, exhaling and being careful about your knees, shoulders, and back are the main considerations. Don't hold your breath while lifting! Always exhale on the concentric portion of the movement. Don't relax the kneecaps at the bottom of a squat or during leg extensions - keep them tight. Push from the heel during squats, and **NEVER** let the knees travel over the toes. Don't let your elbows go much lower than the bench on chest presses. The best way to protect your back is to keep your abs tight and the spine relatively straight (natural curvatures intact). Never lift and twist at the same time.

Resistance also means working against the weight of your own body. Part of being strong is the ability to push and pull your own weight. So include exercises like push-ups, pull-ups (even if you can only hang from the bar initially), and dips in your routine.

Women who do resistance training don't "bulk up." Muscle is far more compact than fat. In females, resistance training makes the muscles toned, longer, and shapely - not bulky - and significantly reduces the risk of osteoporosis. When performed at a proper level, this type of training can also cause major increases in the strength of older individuals.

Ladies... think about this. Body fat takes up five times more space than muscle tissue! Yet muscle burns over 10 times more calories than body fat - 50 vs. 4 calories per day!

3. Water

This aspect of physique transformation is truly overlooked. Look at a whole cantaloupe and two plums.

Now look at four little sugar-free cookies. ***Both choices have the same number of calories!***

Look at a ***huge*** bowl of salad including lettuce, tomatoes, green peppers, cucumbers, carrots, celery, and fat-free dressing (for Pete's sake, not Caesar!!). Now look at a small buttered dinner roll. ***Both have the same number of calories!***

Look at two hearty bowls of Cambell's Chunky soup (say, cheese tortellini with chicken and vegetables) or Campbells Select soup (say, roasted chicken with long grain & wild rice), each made with about a half can of water to add volume. Now look at a small snack-size bag of potato chips. ***Again, both have the same number of calories!***

The fact is that you can have a great, filling, healthful nutrition plan with a very limited calorie budget, so long as you choose to include a lot of foods that naturally have water and fiber content. Don't underestimate the power of whole fruits, salads, meal replacement shakes, and water-based (not oily or cream-based) soups as components of a successful weight loss plan!

Whatever else you drink, adequate water intake is also important to support your metabolism. There is no exact figure, but 8-12 glasses a day of clear, plain water is widely agreed upon (more if you tend to lose a lot of water because of perspiration or hot weather).

4. Four to Six Limited, Balanced Meals Each Day

Regarding what you eat, the key to fitness is balanced nutrition and stable blood sugar. Balanced nutrition means eating protein (preferably between 0.5 and 1 gram per pound of target body weight daily), "clean" carbohydrates, and yes, even some fat.

> A good rule of thumb for weight loss is to multiply your target weight by 9-11 calories per pound daily. Few people will get good fat loss results on fewer than 8, or greater than 12, daily calories per pound of desired weight.
>
> If you're regularly training with weights and want muscle gain without fat loss at all, a target of 15-17 calories per day is about right.

And yes, it is possible to gain muscle and lose fat at the same time (nothing prevents anabolic and catabolic processes from taking place in different cells of the same body).

Be careful about which foods you eat, and how much, in order to fuel your metabolism, promote muscle strength, and maximize fat burning. Ideally, you should eat 5-6 relatively small meals a day. A meal means a limited portion of lean protein (not always meat - egg protein, whey, soy protein and cottage cheese are all great lower-fat alternatives) and a portion of "low-glycemic" carbohydrates (these are generally attached to fiber, so they don't spike your blood sugar, and include oatmeal, whole grains, and whole fruit, as opposed to highly processed carbs like white flour, white rice, and juice). Including fibrous vegetables will also help your digestion, particularly if you're using meal-replacement shakes frequently.

As a side note, the kernel of truth in the Atkins diet is that it's very hard to lose fat if you regularly spike your blood sugar. The danger in the Atkins diet (aside from the dietary fat) is that carbohydrate restriction causes muscle loss and dehydration (which people are very glad to see if they only focus on the scale instead of the source of the weight loss). Choose low glycemic carbs, and you get the best of both worlds - stable blood sugar without compromising muscle tissue.

The goal is to keep a constant nutrient stream and stable blood sugar throughout the day. This kind of nutrition plan maximizes both muscle recovery and fat loss. Again, if your main goal is fat loss, you have to frequently remind yourself that balanced, frequent meals will not help you unless they're also carefully limited in size.

Since the word "meal" frequently makes people think of a large plate of food, or several courses, I to be very clear right now. A "meal" is ***limited portions*** of protein, carbohydrate and fat.

How much is a "limited portion?" If you cup one hand completely over the other, the correct amount of protein or carbohydrate (e.g. chicken, tuna, dry brown rice *before* steaming, dry oatmeal before boiling) will fit completely inside. A flat portion of lean meat might be about the size and thickness of a deck of cards.

Don't get crazy with all this. The main idea is to stick with low glycemic carbs, limit fat intake, carefully monitor portion size and include a lot of water, both as a beverage and within the food itself. You can lose fat without being hungry if you do that. It works!

5. Focus on Creating a Deficit

If your goal is fat loss, your success is not determined by how many calories you burn, nor by how few calories you take in. ***Your fat loss is determined by the difference between these two.*** This difference is called the caloric deficit (or caloric surplus if you're taking in more than you burn). Hands down, the main reason people fail to lose fat on a workout program is that they lose sight of the deficit. They focus, for instance, on increasing their workouts. But then they let their meals creep up in serving size. They think that because they're eating "good" food, they don't need to monitor how much. And in a single binge day, they often blow a good 2 or 3 days of accumulated deficits. Focus on creating the deficit, not intake or output.

Again, this is crucial. If you want to lose fat, you have to burn more calories than you take in, day after day after day. Cardiovascular activity (interval training), building muscle, and other exercise will help you burn calories. Focusing on limited portions and water-based, low-glycemic foods will help you limit your intake while keeping your blood sugar stable. If you let either of these slip, you'll waste your time. If you keep your activity up and your intake down, you'll get fast results.

Think you're good at counting calories?

NEWS ALERT: *Most people are terrible at counting calories!* So you'd better read labels, use measuring cups at least in the beginning, avoid snacking... the whole nine yards. Measure your portions in some way, or they'll creep up in size over time.

Again, a good rule of thumb for fat loss is to multiply your target weight by 9-11 calories per pound daily. Few people will get good fat loss results on less than 8 or more than 12 daily calories per pound of target weight.

IMPORTANT RULE: Never eat less than 1,100 calories per day, regardless of what your goal weight is!

If you're eating far too few calories, you will lose weight. It's just that part of that will be muscle mass and water, and you'll slow your thyroid. If you're not losing weight on the scale, you're either eating enough (and building muscle) or too much (and not losing fat).

Small errors matter, especially if you repeat them day after day. To lose fat, you absolutely must say "no!" to small snacks, instead of "aw, what the heck." Get tough about portion size. **Realize that an extra 20 minutes of cardiovascular exercise is completely wiped out by**

a couple hundred calories of unplanned or excessive eating. When you're tempted to eat that extra snack at night, realize that you may be wiping out the entire day's deficit. If you must eat, grab an apple - not "dry" carbs (pretzels, crackers, chips) or fats. When you're tempted to binge on an off-day well after you're full, you may be wiping out days of progress. Be careful and grab a pear.

6. Sufficient Rest

If you try to transform your physique while depriving yourself of sleep, you're working against yourself. Sleep deprivation causes significant imbalances in several hormones - cortisol, ghrelin, and leptin - and will increase your appetite for junk carbohydrates, reduce your metabolic activity during waking hours, and impede muscle growth. Ideally, find a way to get 8 and preferably 9 hours of sleep a night during the main "transformation" part of your program.

Poor sleep habits will lower the amount of energy you burn each day without you ever being aware of it. Even strolling around or light activity like playing the piano burns 50 or 60 calories more per hour than just sitting. ***You actually burn more calories sleeping than watching TV!*** If you're sleep deprived, you'll do a lot of sitting and TV watching. Your brain also burns about 20% of your total calories a day. Miss a lot of sleep, and you'll reduce that activity too because you'll be less alert.

Physically, most of the physique transformation changes happen while you sleep. **If you don't rest, you don't change.** Repeated lack of rest will also tempt you to miss workouts, crash your energy levels, and interfere with hormones that regulate muscle growth, metabolism, and appetite.

One more time.

Here are the six keys to fast fitness:

1. Cardiovascular exercise (2-4 x weekly, 30-45 minutes per session) - Interval training

2. Resistance training (2-5 x weekly, 25-45 minutes per session)

3. Water!

4. Four to six limited, balanced meals each day

5. Focus on creating a deficit

6. Sufficient rest

I know… I know.

All of this advice means that you'll need some discipline. That's right! But you've got to understand that your body is the way it is right now, because that's how it has adapted to the lifestyle you're living. If you want to change your body, you've also got to change your lifestyle by finding more constructive ways to adapt to your circumstances.

If there's one thing that will create fast fitness and a major physique transformation, it is to follow a complete and integrated program.

REMEMBER: The one key thing is *everything*. You won't get fit by exercising more if you're ignoring your nutrition. You won't get fit by dieting if you're skipping workouts. Don't look for a single trick or technique to be the magic answer, but taken together, these seven elements will create the right environment for fast results.

I think I can!
I think I can!
I think I can!
I think I can!
I think I can!
I think I can!
I think I can!
I think I can!
I know I can!
I think I can!
I think I can!
I think I can!

Positive
thinking
is half
the work...

Chapter 10

The Importance of Core Strength

MANY OF US ARE well accustomed to the development of the glory muscles. Muscles like the chest, shoulders, quads and glutes will always get special attention in the gym - but how many people train their core correctly?

Yes, you see others doing simple exercises like leg raises and crunches to work their "abs," but when we say core, we mean something different.

Think of the core as an entire muscular system that spans the entire surface of the stomach and back. The core is a system of muscles that starts at the hips and runs up to the ribcage - supporting the body the entire way without fault.

With that said, many people have a very weak core which can lead to back pain, hip pain, and even pain in the upper back and neck.

Training your core is important for these main reasons:

1. Your core is your stability. Whenever you're doing an exercise where a load is placed on your back, shoulders, or overhead, your core is the main muscular system that is providing stability.

- **Think of it as the bridge between your upper and lower body.** If the bridge is weak, the connection between the two (upper and lower body) will not be nearly as effective as it could be. Training your core is important for stability in your big overhead movements.

- A weak core means a weak squat and a weak overhead press. If you're a strength athlete, this is something you need to look for.

2. Your core helps you run. Since the core links the upper and lower body together, it will act as a synergist in nearly every step. A strong core means a strong and efficient runner.

- The core will also help to absorb shock. When you're running, your body is impacted with about 40 x your bodyweight on each stride.

- **If your goal is to run a long distance, you must have a strong core.**

3. A strong core makes you look great. Last but not least, the core is important because a strong core looks great. Your core is very important to your overall wellbeing, but training the core for strength and physique is also important.

Having a great core is more diet than training, but when both of these ideas meet in harmony, you'll have a core that is built for strength and success in any setting.

Core Strength - A Crucial Element

Core strength is important for your balance, stability, body strength, weightlifting goals, and running goals. This core muscle system appeals in the aesthetics of training. Plus, it helps keep your back, neck, and hips pain-free.

This is one system that cannot go unnoticed in your training program.

For best results, be sure to try training your core for about 60 minutes of training each week. Dedicated abdominal sessions, rather than 5 minutes after each workout, also seem to show better strength returns.

The best timc to pair core work is at the end of a leg training session. Pair your core training with all your leg workouts and watch as you grow stronger in the core and every aspect of fitness that comes with it.

Start training for core strength today. You'll like the way you feel!

Chapter 11

Combat Fat

13 Untold Ultra-Fat Burning Secrets

I'M SURE YOU'VE SEEN hundreds of other fat loss "secret" tips out there. They all say pretty much the same thing. Eat every 2-3 hours, drink plenty of water, avoid white flour, don't eat refined sugar, don't order dessert, don't drink soda, use your fist to determine portion size, do cardio 30 to 60 minutes and build more lean muscle to speed up metabolism.

Those are all great tips, but they are definitely not worthy being called untold ultra-fat burning secrets.

I have personally witnessed hundreds of my clients kick 20 pounds to the curb and get a six-pack in 8 weeks using the exact information that I am about to share with you.

This fat melting knowledge has literally taken me 10 years of research and volunteering my own body as a guinea pig to perfect it. And now, here it is, for you – FREE!

Fat-Loss Secret #1

The #1 make or break success factor is getting your mindset right! Looking back over the last ten years at my clients who have had the most Jaw Dropping, Eye Popping Extreme results, and they all had a certain mind set before every workout. No, they didn't put on war paint and go commando (well, some of them did). Simply put, before every workout, they committed to giving 100%. No excuses. No complaining. Believe it or not, once you practice this mindset a few times, it becomes an easy habit.

- **Mindset tip** – before each workout, visualize what is most important to you. Being healthy for your kids, looking ripped at the beach, having girls want your body, being the hottest girl at the club, etc. Picture what inspires you and say to yourself - that's me, that's me, that's me...

Fat-Loss Secret #2

Technically, this does not burn fat, but it will make your waist look slimmer instantly. As I look around, I see endless clients with poor posture, which results from training programs which overly concentrates on working the chest and shoulders, combined with sedentary jobs where you are sitting at a desk or in front of a computer terminal all day. The result of this poor posture is rounded shoulders, and a slumped forward appearance, which just pushes your belly out! To test this, all you have to do is stand up straight while drawing your shoulders back and instantly witness your stomach flatten. Strengthening the muscles responsible for maintaining an upright posture (lower back) and drawing your shoulders back (scapula retractors) will lead to a flattening effect on your stomach. Another quick remedy for bad posture is stretching your chest muscles.

- **Tip** - A great posture improving and waist slimming exercise is "seated rows." Sit up straight, extend arms forward all the way, pull back with your elbows against your sides and squeeze shoulder together.

Fat-Loss Secret #3

Unless you want to spend hours and hours in the gym, have a fast-paced workout. Most people don't have all day to work out (I sure don't). By not resting in-between exercises, you can build muscle and burn fat at the same time. I have personally tested this by putting a heart rate monitor on clients and comparing a fast-paced, intense weight workout vs. taking a spin class. It was shocking to discover that they actually got more cardio in the fast-paced weight workout than in the spin class. What could be better than saving time and melting more fat?

- **Tip** – Maintain a vigorous pace. Keep moving from excrcise to exercise. One trick is to bring a pair of dumbbells next to a treadmill. Run for 60 seconds on the treadmill, then jump off and do a dumbbell exercise, then get back on the treadmill. Keep alternating throughout the workout.

- **Tip** - Plan your workouts ahead of time. Don't waste time and let your heart rate go down trying to think of what to do next. Spending a little time planning your workouts will save you a lot of time and yield better results in the long run.

- **Tip** - Pick exercises that do not require a lot of time to set up. It's all about pace and saving time.

- Exercises that take more than a few seconds to set up let your heart rate go down and can add a lot of extra time to your workout.

- **Tip** - Keep your routine flexible. If a piece of equipment that you need to use is occupied, don't wait or ask to work in. Just move on to the next exercise and come back later. Keep the pace going and the fat melting.

Fat-Loss Secret #4

Use "free" snacks and drinks that fill you up, curb your cravings, but won't add any significant extra calories. Eat and drink as many of these free snacks and drinks as you want.

- **Tip** – When you get the late night sweet tooth, try a delicious homemade Chai Tea. This is how I make it. Put two Yogi Mayan Cocoa Spice tea bags in a cup (I use a big 20 ceramic cup) of boiling water. Add a tiny dash (it's very sweet) of KAL brand Stevia. Let it steep for a few minutes then add some No-Sugar added Silk Soy Milk.

- **Tip** – Cut up cucumber, Jicama or celery. Munch away all you want!

Fat-Loss Secret #5

Don't just work out aimlessly. Take pictures, measurements, and weigh yourself before your next workout (or your first workout if you're just getting started) then set a goal and a date, usually 6 to 8 weeks. If you can, get someone to agree to do the measurements to help keep you accountable. Over the years, I discovered that when clients know they are going to get measured for progress on a certain date, they are less likely to miss workouts or cheat on their eating.

- **Tip** – set a realistic goal so that you stay motivated and do not get discouraged.

Fat-Loss Secret #6

A big secret to melting fat is to do exercises that work several muscles at once. This is important for two reasons:

1. Working several muscles at once burns more calories because it requires your heart to work harder to supply oxygen to the areas under stress.

2. It saves you time.

Your workouts take a lot less time because you don't have to do separate exercises for each muscle. You won't see these super fat burning exercises too often at your local gym because most people just don't know about them and their fat-crushing benefits.

- **Tip** – Do Dumbbell Squat Presses: Target = Butt, Thighs, Shoulders, Triceps, and Cardio

Hold dumbbells level with ears in the press position. Squat down until thighs are parallel to the floor. Stand back up and then press dumbbells over your head. Lower them back down and repeat 20 to 30 times.

- **Tip** – Do Walking Lunge Lateral Raise Curls: Target = Butt, Thighs, Shoulders, Biceps, Triceps, and Cardio

With dumbbells at your sides, lunge forward with your left leg, then bring your right foot forward up to your left foot. Next, Raise the dumbbells laterally out to your sides until they are level with your ears, and then lower them back to your sides. Next, curl the dumbbells up and down with your palms up. Repeat, alternating legs, until 20 to 30 lateral raise curls are performed.

- **Tip** – Do Burpee Pushups: Target = Butt,

Thighs, Shoulders, Triceps Chest, Core and Cardio

Do one push up. Quickly jump feet forward to a squatting position. Jump high into the air, raising your hands above your head. Land with feet shoulder width apart, on the balls of your feet and drop back into a squat. Jump feet back to a pushup position. Repeat 20 to 30 times in a fluid motion.

Fat-Loss Secret #7

Don't work your abs... That's right, I said it! Abdominal exercises do not burn fat away from your abs! I see so many people every day in the gym wasting their time crunching away, then wondering why their body hasn't changed after months.

- **Tip** – you can incorporate a few stomach exercises like hanging leg raises and cable twists between exercises as part of your fast-paced workout.

Fat-Loss Secret #8

Eat real food to get lean! Ever watch The Discovery Channel? See the tribes in the jungle. You never see anyone who is fat, even the elders have six-packs. Why? They eat real food and stay active.

Stay away from processed foods. The food companies strip out the good stuff like fiber and nutrients.

What you have left is food that has way more calories than normal. Plus, the worst part is that they are high glycemic, which means your body treats it like sugar. The good news is once you cut out these processed foods for a couple weeks, you lose your cravings. I'm not saying to not have a life. I eat burgers, pizza or have a piece of cake from time to time.

- **Tip** – watch out for foods and drinks that people think are "healthy" like bagels, pretzels and sports drinks like vitamin water. Consuming these is like eating table sugar.

- **Tip** – Stick to foods like lean meat and fish, long-grain brown rice, and fruits and vegetables.

Fat-Loss Secret #9

Alkalizing the body sheds fat fast! The body is naturally acidic. However, the foods we eat add to this acidity and the fat in our body stores the additional acid, which results in overweight problems and an unhealthy body. To protect against acid buildup, the body begins to create and store fat. Even if you are on a weight-loss diet and you exercise, your body will try to hold on to this fat because it is important for protection against acids. That is why many people whom restore alkalinity in their body find it incredibly easier to lose weight.

There are certain foods that are alkaline and help to flush the acid and fat from the body.

- **Tip** – Most green vegetables are high alkaline. Some really high acid foods are: Fast food, milk, eggs, cream, cheese, pork and red meat.

Fat-Loss Secret #10

Be prepared. Most of the time, clients eat poorly because they did not bring food with them or did not prepare. Bring healthy snacks with you like apples and almonds. If you can, bring some Tupperware containers with healthy meals. Keep it simple. If you don't feel like bringing food, then plan out some healthy restaurants or stores that you can patronize.

- **Tip** – Get a rice cooker and keep some long-grain brown basmati rice cooking on your counter. Also, pre-cook some chicken or fish. It will only take a few minutes to prepare 1 or 2 meals and grab a few snacks to bring with you.

Fat-Loss Secret #11

Warning: Artificially Sweetened "Sugar Free" Foods Make You FAT. Did you know that most foods labeled as "sugar free" or "low-carb" actually contain artificial sweeteners, sugar alcohols, and other additives that create a hormonal disaster inside your body, actually causing your body to STORE more belly fat and increase cravings! Also, foods labeled "whole grain" only have to contain a small fraction of whole grains, where the majority can still be refined starches and sugars that spike your blood sugar faster than a bowl of ice cream.

- **Tip** – Stop eating foods with artificial sweeteners for two weeks, then try it again. It will taste like disgusting sweet chemicals.

- **Tip** - If you really want to sweeten something, use an all-natural sugar free sweetener like Stevia or Xilatol.

Fat-Loss Secret #12

Don't cheat on your nutrition plan for 21 days. It takes the brain 21 days to reset itself and create a new habit. When you want to make a change, don't tell yourself you are doing it for life; tell yourself that you are going to try it for 21 days. Now, when you have completed this for 21 days, your conscious mind has the choice of stopping it or carrying on, or so it thinks. Your neural pathways have formed already and you will more than likely continue with your new habit. You will have seen thc benefits along the way your unconscious will want to continue if it has been beneficial.

- **Tip** – Make it as easy as possible for you to have a successful 21 days. Use your day planner to schedule eating and workout times. Leave reminder notes to yourself.

- **Tip** – Try working out first thing in the morning before your busy day starts and your workout gets put on the back burner.

Fat-Loss Secret #13

For at least one week, write down everything you eat and drink. You have to write it down right before the food or drink is consumed. By writing it down first, you will have a moment to stop and think about whether this decision is going to melt belly fat or pack it on.

- **Tip** – Have someone agree to review your food journal every day. Make an agreement that for each day you do not give him your journal, you owe him $10.00 and every time you cheat you owe $1.00 dollar. Doing this will help keep you accountable.

Fat-Loss Secret #14 *BONUS TIP*

Time after time, I see so many people with good intentions lace up their gym shoes, put on their workout clothes, arrive at the gym, realize they aren't sure of what exercises to do, how many reps, how much weight, the proper form, how often and then get discouraged and just go home. Oh, and of course, lose the motivation to stick to their nutrition plan as well.

- **Tip** – Spend months or years becoming a health

and fitness expert, or go to a professional Fitness & Medical Facility that'll help you melt the belly fat and build a firm-toned body… like Bopp Optimal Health, where you can jumpstart your health and fitness journey, and discover why we have so many walking, talking billboards (aka satisfied patients singing praise about us) who will happily tell you about their success stories since joining our Bopp Optimal Health family. Call us at 318- 550-0050, and we'll be happy to help you start your health and fitness journey.

Thank you for taking the time out of your schedule to read this special report. If you know anyone on this planet who would love to get their hands on this body-transforming information, (it could be a friend, family member, co-worker or anyone else that you know), please feel free to tell them about this book.

Better yet… Buy a copy and send it to them as a gift! They will thank you and so will I.

Chapter 12

52 Ways To Lose A Pound A Week

You can achieve weight-loss and keep it off forever.

How can I be so sure?

Besides mountains of research from leading experts, there are thousands of readers and/or clients of my **Small Steps Every Day** program who have successfully done it. Over the years, their letters and e-mails have been filled with practical tips, as well as the pride and pleasure of people who feel great about themselves. They can run, jump, play on the floor with the kids, wear sexy clothes — newly empowered to do whatever they want.

That's why I decided to create this book for you, a collection of stories and successful strategies for permanent weight loss.

Here are some useful tips that will inspire you:

Believe in yourself

1. Ditch all-or-nothing thinking. Every time that Sandra Wadsworth, 41, attempted weight loss, she'd quit at the first slip up. *"But I finally lost 20 pounds when my weight-loss specialist helped me see that I wasn't a bad person. Everyone makes mistakes. The key is to learn from them."*

2. Start with a bang. At 315 pounds, Heidi Feick had long hidden behind her blond, waist-length hair. But when she decided to take a risk and cut it, her courage to change sparked a sense of purpose and commitment. Feick, 32, began eating healthier and walking every day. In one year, she dropped from a size 30 to a size 4. Pounds lost: 185.

3. Seize your strength. *"I stopped telling myself that I was destined to be overweight forever,"* says Adrienne Sussman, 52. *"I accepted that whatever was broken, I had the power to fix."* To get comfortable with yourself, stand in front of a mirror completely naked every couple of weeks. Find one body part that you like — even if it's your elbows! When Sussman stopped berating herself, she shed 30 pounds.

4. Make a dream book. *"Before I could change my body, I had to change my thinking,"* recalls Sonia Turner, 43. *"To build my confidence, I created a scrapbook of people exercising and overcoming adversity. I included a photo of my husband's company Christmas party. I'd always stayed home because I was embarrassed, but I announced, 'Next year, we're going.'"* When the holidays rolled around, Turner had lost 135 pounds. She and her husband danced the night away.

5. See a pro. At age 50, George Trott was diagnosed with diabetes and heart disease. That news got him to trim down 40 pounds, but he needed to lose more. On the suggestion of his daughter, he visited a dietitian who helped him fine-tune his diet and a personal trainer who helped him fine-tune his activities. He finally shed all the necessary pounds, and his subsequent blood tests improved, too.

By the way... I'm more than happy to help you get everything in place, and getting you that health and fit body. You'll do even better with me leading the way. If you'd like me to help, reach out to me by going to **(318) 550-0050**.

6. Be flexible. Kris Roberts' schedule didn't allow her to set up a rigid exercise routine. So Roberts, 37, took a different approach. *"I did whatever was most convenient. My only goal was to do something to raise my heart rate and work up a sweat every day — even if only for five minutes."* Her flexibility kept Roberts motivated to exercise and enjoy it. She's maintained her 50-pound weight loss for 10 years.

7. Don't blame it on age. Connie Bissonnette, 58, had given up, believing that weight gain was a normal part of aging. Her son proved her wrong. *"He said, 'Just give me 10 minutes, three times a week,'"* Bissonnette recalls. *"He devised a workout of exercises such as seated leg lifts and wall push-ups that I did at home."* Bissonnette began enjoying the exercises and eventually worked her way up to a 30-minute routine. Pounds lost: 41.

8. Step away from the scale. By the time Kym Hubert's weight reached 245, the 41-year-old was checking her scale three times a day. Desperate to help, her husband smashed the scale. *"It was depressing having my 'addiction' taken away,"* she says. But she started focusing on a new weight loss interest: walking. When Hubert finally weighed herself a year later, she'd lost 80 pounds.

9. Personalize your plan. Dozens of weight loss plans had failed Lisa Douglass, 29, so she created her own. *"I decided to be responsible for my choices,"* she says. Douglass scoured exercise and nutrition materials, chose the best advice, and developed her own program. She went from 280 pounds to 160 over a two-year period. *"Even though I still make bad choices occasionally, I like the fact that I'm making them,"* she says.

Set the right goals

10. Build on success. More than 10 years ago, Marlene Dropp, 54, took her first walk around the block in an effort to lose some of her 200 pounds. She set a goal of five miles a day. When she achieved that landmark within two months, she came up with a new goal: to cover a mile in 13 minutes. She did that easily and lost 50 pounds in two years. Then Dropp began entering racewalking competitions — and had the thrill of completing a marathon for her 51st birthday.

11. Use a symbol. Dinah Burnette, 38, hung an expensive black dress on her closet door. At 245 pounds, she couldn't even pull it over her hips. *"I tried it on every four weeks. When I eventually got in it, the buttons were four feet apart!"* she laughs. One year later and 100 pounds lighter, she fit into the size 12 with room to spare. Ten years later, Burnette still keeps her size 24 dress in the closet as a reminder.

Eat more

12. Move to eat. Rick Dyers' choice was this: Eat fewer calories, or burn more with exercise. He chose the latter and took off more than 50 pounds. In the beginning, Dyers, 46, could barely walk for 15 minutes at a time. Now he runs about one hour every day, covering roughly seven miles. *"I switched from walking to running to burn even more calories,"* he says.

13. Fill up. A 50-year battle of the bulge ended when Helen Stein, 73, admitted her love of eating. Instead of cutting down, she eats large salads, big pink grapefruits, whole cantaloupes, and big chunks of watermelon. These make her feel full without the fat or calories piling up. And Stein hasn't regained an ounce of the 38 pounds that she lost 15 years ago.

14. Seduce your taste buds. When Alice Layne, 42, traded in pizza for international cuisine, she lost 67 pounds and four dress sizes. "The new tastes transformed my palate."

15. Get it fresh. Carla Tuckerton, 44, stopped having headaches and lost 20 pounds when she gave up highly processed foods. *"Almost everything I ate was processed and loaded with artificial sweeteners or salt. I was practically living on frozen dinners, diet sodas, and sugar- free desserts."*

Now Tuckerton buys fish and chicken from a farmers' market, shops for organically grown fruits and veggies, and cooks her own meals. Spring water with a slice of lemon has replaced colas, and she drinks her tea unsweetened.

16. Don't start empty. Susan Carlson, 42, always chose an extra 15 minutes of sleep over a bowl of cereal, until her slim friends advised her to eat breakfast. She started slowly with a slice of toast and a cup of coffee, gradually adding a bowl of cold or hot cereal. Her lunches got smaller, and she stopped snacking on cookies and chips in the afternoon. Pounds lost: 36.

17. Earmark "occasion" foods. Rosemary Chiaverini, 50, lost 87 pounds when she began linking eating to special events. She eats hamburgers and hot dogs only at picnics, popcorn only at the movies, and pasta only on theater nights. *"I tie my eating to the ambience of what I'm doing.*

It gives the food extra meaning," she says. It also gives Chiaverini license to indulge without going overboard.

18. Snack on cereal. Teresa Pucsek's weight loss stalled because of her apple strudel, a favorite treat that reminded her of her childhood in Hungary. *"I had to figure out a way to eat differently but still get that familiar 'old home' feeling,"* says the 80-year-old. Her solution: sweetened cereal. The sugar satisfies her sweet tooth, and the milk reminds her of her childhood. This satisfying, lower-calorie snack has helped her maintain an 86-pound weight loss for 24 years.

Eat smart

19. Dine alone. Debbee Sereduck, 38, dropped an astounding 234 pounds when, after preparing dinner for her family, she started taking hers into the living room and didn't return until everything in the kitchen was completely put away. *"This kept me from taking extra helpings or finishing the kids' uneaten food,"* says Sereduck. *"It also gave me a little quiet time."*

20. Create "The End." Linda O'Hanlon, 30, never got the "full" signal that makes most people push away their plates. *"When I sat down for a spaghetti dinner, I didn't* *get up until every last strand was gone,"* she says. Instead of relying on her stomach, O'Hanlon decided to start measuring her portions. After her brain took charge, she proceeded to drop three pants sizes. Two years later, O'Hanlon's holding steady at 151 pounds and now can eyeball her portions.

21. Read the box. Phyllis Barbour, 70, ate all the right weight loss foods, worked out three or four times a week, and was on her feet constantly. So she was puzzled when her clothes started feeling a bit snug. Then Barbour picked up a package of her beloved bagels and read the nutrition label. One of those big, doughy delectables equaled four servings of bread. When she checked other labels, she found more of the same. *"I saw an immediate difference when I started paying closer attention to serving sizes,"* she says. Pounds lost: 7.

22. Check your fluids. For Lent, Jim Gorman, 33, substituted water and club soda for sugary beverages and alcohol. By Easter, 40 days later, he was 20 pounds lighter.

23. Switch your plate. Eating less wasn't easy for Gretchen Harvey, 32, until she substituted a salad plate for a dinner plate. (The former holds only about 60 percent of the amount of food.) "I was still seeing a full plate of food, so psychologically it didn't seem that I was denying myself anything," she says. Harvey lost 30 pounds.

Get moving

24. Use nervous energy. When you're under stress, your body releases adrenaline in anticipation of either fighting or fleeing. But in combating everyday stress, that biological response can urge you to eat. When Robert Kim, 36, took up running to deal with pressure, he lost 45 pounds.

25. Breathe, don't gasp. Lisa Kay Wojcik, 33, was so overweight and out of shape that two minutes' worth of low-impact aerobics left her so breathless that she called 911. A doctor at the hospital told her that she was breathing incorrectly. *"He told me to breathe in through my nose and out through my mouth while exercising, and to exhale harder to force a deeper inhale. This sends more oxygen to the muscles."* Two years later, Wojcik had lost 215 pounds and gone from a size 36 to a size 2.

26. Catch up on reading. Books on tape helped Rebecca Harding, 49, run off 68 pounds and keep it off for 15 years. *"I played the tapes only when I was running,"* she says. *"Recently, when I ran to a tape of "The Horse Whisperer," I went almost nine miles up a steep hill in the rain!"*

27. Stretch out. At 220 pounds, Melissa MacKinnon, 33, decided to try yoga. *"It looked so relaxing and easy, so perfect for my imperfect body,"* she says. MacKinnon's energy level soared, and as she became more attuned to her body, she began to crave vegetables, not chocolate. She replaced refined sugars with whole grains. *"As yoga rewired my mind, I learned to take better care of my body,"* she says. MacKinnon's held to her 60-pound weight loss for seven years.

28. Get out. Sharon Evans, 38, got involved in orienteering (a sport where you find your way using only a compass and a map) to improve her navigational skills for backpacking. Being out in the fresh air replaced eating in front of the TV. As her orienteering skills grew, her waistline shrank. Pounds lost: 20.

29. Phone-ercise. When Jeri Jefferis, now 57, left her job as a physical education instructor, she worried about regaining the 30 pounds she had lost earlier. With two small children, she was hard-pressed to find time to work out. Then she realized that chatting with friends, listening to phone solicitations, even being put on hold were opportunities to keep in shape. *"Sometimes I'd simply pace the floor. Other times, I'd do squats or leg lifts. If I hadn't started doing that, I know I'd have a weight problem today."*

30. Act out. Kirie Pedersen's job was making her fat. *"Virtually every day for six years, I was glued to a chair,"* says the 48-year-old. Pedersen began stretching in the morning. She swung her arms vigorously when she walked. *"I'd also set a timer to go off every hour,"* she says. *"That was my cue: For 15 minutes, I'd squat, skip, wiggle, dance — whatever I felt like doing — just like kids do."* A year later, Pedersen was 40 pounds slimmer, wearing a size six instead of a 14.

Build muscle

31. Be an active sitter. Lynn Oatman, 48, doesn't relax when she sits down. She hoists a pair of dumbbells up and down for about half an hour while watching TV. *"I've gone from somebody who could barely lift a 10-pound bag of potatoes to bench-pressing 75 pounds. It makes me feel powerful,"* she boasts. Oatman has dropped 60 pounds in two years.

32. Shape a new body. Watching a bodybuilding competition on TV 20 years ago spurred Sharon Turrentine — who had not exercised in years — to head for the gym. *"Five pounds was the most that I could lift when I started,"* recalls Turrentine, 55. *"Now I bench-press more than 100 pounds."*

Within 3 years, Turrentine dropped four dress sizes. The person who'd once undressed in her closet decided to show off her 5'2", 109-pound body in competition. Over the years, she's brought home 15 trophies.

Binge-proof your life

33. Pop in some inspiration. Marcia Carter, 41, avoided temptations — and lost 35 pounds — by keeping motivational tapes and books handy. *"If I was near a fast-food drive-through, I'd pop a tape into my car stereo,"* she says. *"The pep talk helped me to stay on track. It also helped when I'd slip and eat something that I shouldn't."*

34. Feel what's gone. Whenever Pat Beyer, 41, gets the urge to splurge, she picks up a 5-pound bag of sugar. *"I've taken off the equivalent of five bags of sugar in weight, and I don't want them back,"* she proclaims.

35. Please your dentist. Thirty-five-year-old Lisa Gardiner's downfall was after-dinner noshing, so she fell back on an old college trick: *"I brush my teeth immediately after dinner. It's my signal that eating is over for the day."* (Toothpaste also alters the flavor of food, so it doesn't taste good.) Pounds lost: 25.

36. Turn in instead of giving in. Cheryl Lachenmayer's weight loss resolve dissolved each evening. To beat her cravings, the 39-year-old went to bed, sometimes as early as 9:00. She also went from 170 pounds to a slim 130.

37. Steep into evening. Feeling tired after work and anticipating the evening's chores made Jeanette Green, 60, anxious and tense. At 300 pounds, she'd head straight for the refrigerator to soothe herself.

"But then I remembered something from Overeaters Anonymous: 'If you get your head straight, your body will follow.'" The next day, Lachenmayer brewed a cup of herbal tea as soon as she walked through the door. Then she curled up to relax and recharge. Her teatime became a treasured ritual and stopped the munchies. She took off 140 pounds and has maintained her weight loss for more than 18 years.

38. Grab a magazine. When the fridge calls Cynthia Herrmann, 48, she picks up a magazine or newspaper. *"If I still feel hungry after reading for 15 minutes, I eat. But I often get so absorbed that 30 minutes fly by, and the craving's gone,"* she says. Pounds lost: 90.

39. Follow the beat. Bingeing was Mark Maron's way to deal with a work crisis, a fight with a loved one, or anything else that made him feel bad.

One day, Maron, 36, decided to skip his usual fast-food place and head for the music store. *"I picked out two CDs, including one featuring my favorite song, 'Born to Be Alive,'"* he recalls. He got so pumped up that he forgot about food and headed for the gym. That habit eventually erased 25 pounds.

Talk yourself thin

40. Carry a pen. *"I was tired of compliments that stopped at my face,"* says Juanita Dillard, a 37-year-old makeup artist who weighed 274 pounds. *"I was constantly surrounded by thin, gorgeous models, and I wanted to be like them."*

Dillard started writing about her stress instead of feeding it. Within a year and a half, she dropped from a size 24 to a size 6. One time, halfway through a binge brought on by the stress of losing her pet, Dillard reached into her purse and felt her journal. Out it came, and she started writing. After putting her feelings down on paper, her desire to eat was gone. *"Journaling has become my no-cal stress buster,"* she says.

41. Announce your intentions. *"The support that I got was unbelievable,"* says Irma Toce, 42. *"Clients and coworkers told me how wonderful I looked. A friend who had always baked cookies agreed to prepare just one special chocolate chip cookie a week for me. On days when I didn't feel like exercising, my eldest stepdaughter would encourage me. And when the weather got cold, my husband bought me a treadmill."* With all that support, Toce easily lost 70 pounds.

42. Dial a friend. Freelance writer Carol Kennedy, 45, got her cravings under control and lost 20 pounds when she and a couple of friends developed a telephone support group. *"When I craved ice cream, I'd call one of my friends. She'd talk me through it and help me stick to my plan,"* Kennedy explains.

43. Stay focused. When David Zimmerman arrived home after a year overseas, he didn't recognize his wife, Hope: She'd lost 121 pounds. *"Aiming to shock him had been a big motivator,"* says Hope, 31. But a snide comment ("She's not as thin as your brother's girlfriend") threatened her success. *"I was devastated by the remark,"* she recalls, *"but I let go of it by focusing on the kindness that I received from others."*

Make motivation easy

44. Revisit the pits. When Beth Linden, who'd lost 100 pounds, slipped back to her old habits and regained 15 pounds, she pulled out the audiotape that documented the worst moment of her life. *"I could hear my voice quiver as I described meeting my daughter's friend, who said, 'I didn't know your mommy was fat.' I hated putting my daughter in such an awkward situation; I felt lonely and empty. I was embarrassed to shop for clothes. I hated myself back then and didn't want to go back there,"* recalls Linden, 39. The tape turned her around and has kept her on the weight loss track for more than five years.

45. Schedule nudges. Bevan Brooks, 22, used a calendar full of motivational "carrots" to shed 20 pounds. *"I would remind myself of parties, trips, sporting events, visitors from out of town, and weddings in the weeks and months ahead,"* she says. *"Every time I'd consider bagging a workout or eating pepperoni pizza, I'd remind myself of an upcoming event. How I looked meant more to me than any piece of pizza."*

46. Take a time-out. *"I relaxed my strict dietary rules on weekends, and I stopped feeling deprived,"* says Helene Gullaksen, 35. *"When a craving hits during the week, I tell myself, 'This isn't the last time I can eat this food,' and it helps me walk away from whatever is tempting me."* Pounds lost: 50.

47. Be blunt (with yourself). Oprah Winfrey and her personal trainer, Bob Greene, inspired 300-pound Tawni Gomes to start exercising when the 34-year-old met Greene at a book signing. *"I heard another woman ask him how she was supposed to find time to exercise with four kids, a house, and a full-time job,"* recalls Gomes. *"Bob looked her straight in the eye and said, 'You're not ready to lose weight.' I was shocked, but realized that I was making identical excuses."*

"Everybody has the same number of hours in a day. If people are busier than I can find time to exercise, so can I." The next morning, Gomes got up early to walk. It was the start of what would become a daily ritual. Pounds lost: 125.

48. Cover the clock. Some nights, Mitch Lipka, 34, could barely look at his stationary bike, let alone ride it. Then he developed the diversionary tactic of throwing a towel or T-shirt over the timer to concentrate on something else. He'd get so lost in thought that the time was up before he even knew it. Now he never misses a session. Pounds lost: 200.

49. Do 10, then switch. Whenever Cheryl Allard, 50, goes to the gym, she uses one machine for 10 minutes, then moves on to something else. This boredom-beating strategy worked so well that Allard started going to the gym six days a week. Within a year, she took off 100 pounds.

50. Showcase "before" photos. Both Julia Ferraro, 37, and her mother, Adelaide, were 5 feet 2 inches tall and weighed 205 pounds. A family picture brought them to tears. *"You can know that you're getting bigger, but it doesn't hit you until you look at a picture of yourself,"* says Julia. Instead of stashing the photo out of sight, they agreed to display it prominently for weight loss motivation. Since that shot was taken, the two have lost a combined 90 pounds and five dress sizes — and they've added a new, beaming mother/ daughter photo to their tabletop gallery.

51. Be your own coach. Jean Ann Pock, 29, had trouble getting up early to walk until she read a quote from legendary football coach Vince Lombardi: *"Winning is not a sometime thing; it's an all-the- time thing."* Says Pock,

"I realized that I had to win every little battle along the way — including the skirmishes with my alarm clock. I had to think like a winner to become one." Now, Pock throws off the covers every morning. Pounds lost: 85.

Reward yourself

52. Celebrate every victory. Susan DeFusco ultimately managed to shed 100 pounds, but day-to-day, she focused on losing just the next 5. Each time she accomplished one of those baby steps, she would reward herself with a bubble bath or an exercise tape. *"You need to look at each 5-pound loss as something worth celebrating,"* advises the 38-year-old.

There you have it! 52 ways to lose a pound a week. Even if you only apply a handful of these suggestions... but do so diligently... you will have tremendous success reaching your weight-loss goal, as well. So, find the strategies you feel comfortable applying to your life... ***and make it happen!***

And if you're not sure where to start, reach out to me and let me help you jumpstart your journey. No risk. No obligation. Just me helping you determine the best plan of action. Feel free to call and chat with me and my team at (318) 550-0050.

Chapter 13

Discipline Your Self-Discipline

T HE GREATEST BODYBUILDING GENES in the world are useless if they are not backed up by self-discipline. The body is inherited at birth; self-discipline is something you acquire. To develop self-discipline, you have to take possession of your mind. Sounds weird, doesn't it? Take possession of something you already own by using it to possess itself. But it's not weird when you look at it closely.

In effect, self-discipline is about control - the ability to control your mind with such strength that your emotions and desires are regulated and managed in any direction you want. In a way, self-discipline is a kind of mental and moral training session. You can develop it, or you can lose it, just like your physical condition. But self-discipline is a lot trickier to maintain, because it involves the need for a harmonious arrangement of the parts. You must balance the emotions of the heart with the reasoning of the mind, and that's always a tough thing to do.

These days, self-discipline is something of a rarity. Most people do not want to be disciplined. They would rather please the first emotion or desire that pops into their head. Bodybuilders are a different breed. Even the average bodybuilder is an absolute expert on weight control when compared to the masses. But that's not saying much. I want you to become a powerful human being. This can happen when you increase your self-discipline. To do that, carefully consider the following points about this valuable feature:

1. Learn from the Leaders. Throughout the ages, all great leaders have one thing in common: they consciously fight against the human tendency toward comfort. Leaders are keenly aware that people follow the weakest part of their own human nature, allowing this to dominate their actions. **Leaders dominate their own human nature.** They resist the urge to be comfortable. They stay hungry. They are constantly challenging themselves instead of succumbing to the easy way. There's a very subtle, but important point here.

The key word is *easy*. Leaders never take it easy. This makes them very special human beings. While all others are choosing the easiest and fastest way to get what they want now, with no thought for secondary consequences, leaders apply their willpower and rise above this weak tendency of humanity.

This natural quality of leaders tells you something about bodybuilding. Every time you put forth an effort in some particular direction, a part of your mind will offer you an easier route. Not more effective, just easier. **Watch for it!** When it happens, fight it and destroy it.

When you start watching out for this seductive mental offer, you strengthen your mind. It may occur while you are dieting. Say nobody's looking around to monitor you, so you go ahead and have that pastry. Your mind says to you, "It's OK. You'll need the extra carbs for your workout, and you won't notice it on your physique, so go ahead!" There's the offer. ***Resist it!***

Even if that piece of pastry may not make a cosmetic difference, it's making a serious difference in your mind. By giving in to the urge, you lower your self-respect; you set yourself up for an easier mark the next time.

If you give in again to another mental "offer," your self-respect will continue to spiral downward, and your self-discipline will weaken as well. Refuse the offer instead! Do what you should do when you should do it, whether you like it or not. Never give in to a passing fancy, whim, or impulse. By resisting, you'll raise your self-respect, and your self-discipline will increase as well. ***That's exactly why people who have great self-respect also have great self-discipline!***

Have you ever sat in a diner and watch overweight people put down all kinds of food? You are seeing poor self-respect in action. It's not a very inspiring thing to see.

Keep in mind that temptations come in a wide variety of formats and in subtle degrees. In the gym, for example, I have seen many people give up long before they should have, simply because it was easier to quit at that point. To the untrained observer, they still look like they are working out. But the truth of the matter is that they are succumbing to the weaker part of their mind.

Conversely, I have seen many people set personal records in a lift when they did not know that extra weight was slipped on the bar before their set. That's because their mind didn't know the weight was added, either. Otherwise, they would have assuredly found a reason to not complete the lift.

Get the quality of leaders -never take it easy. Be on the lookout for these enticing "offers." Turn them down when they show up, and your self-discipline will grow.

2. Delay Gratification. Having self-discipline doesn't mean that you deprive yourself of pleasures or that you can't have fun. It simply means that you delay the fun whenever necessary. For example, let's say you've just finished watching a movie with some friends, and they suggest going out to a restaurant.

Knowing that you have a leg workout tomorrow, you decline because it'll take two hours out of your sleep time. If it were a day off for you, then you'd accept the offer. Sounds simple enough, but it's surprising how many bodybuilders try to get the best of both worlds, only to end up losing.

Furthering the example, you decide to go to the restaurant, and within minutes, you are having a great time. Although your original intention was to go for only half an hour, a quick glance at your watch reveals that you have blown two hours. You rush home to get to sleep, but the next day your leg workout suffers, anyway. You had to go light because your strength wasn't there. As you can see, those were a very critical two hours. But you weren't thinking about them when you were laughing and joking at the restaurant.

Never make the mistake of serving two masters. You'll only end up serving one, at the cost of the other. Delaying gratification is an all-or-nothing proposition, not a halfway measure.

Also, don't fall into the trap of believing you're missing out on all the fun. I have two things to tell you about that ridiculous notion. First of all, where is all of this fun? In a bar? If you think so, then go to one. You will encounter loads of out-of-shape, overweight people who smoke and drink and talk a lot but say things of little substance. That's a bar. They typically are depressing environments crammed full of people who wouldn't even think for one moment to delay gratification. They want it all now. They've got it, all right. But they don't have great bodies, healthy lungs, or good nutrition flowing through them. What they have is not much in a way of a healthy lifestyle. If they did, you wouldn't catch them in a bar.

Second, do you think fun is whatever your friends happen to be doing while you're not there? Phone them from where you are, and you'll see that not really much is going on. They are probably just standing around and talking. Not much more than that. I'm not trying to condemn the whole process of socializing. Of course, it's necessary, and it should be done.

The main point is that you're not missing out on all that fun. Those people in the bar would love to look like you. They think you look like fun. The whole idea of missing out on all the action is a myth. There is plenty of time for you to do whatever you want. You just have to know when to delay gratification. Believe me; ***the fun will be all yours in the end!***

3. Follow Through. Discipline yourself to persist. It builds character. Character is the ability to follow through after the enthusiasm and emotion that started your resolution has passed.

Regardless of how much passion you have - and I advocate that you have a lot - there will be times when everything seems to get you down. This is normal. The only people who are "up" 100% of the time are brainwashed people who belong to cults.

It is expected now and then that you feel that somehow all of your efforts are feeble and your actions inconsequential.

However, it's also true that these states are transitory. They last briefly, and they're gone.

We are emotional creatures, and as such, we will waver now and then. Don't be too hard on yourself when you hit a temporary low spot. **The main point is to remember to keep on going.** Don't let these little backslides stop you. All they did is just put a few extra hours between you and your goals.

When you've made a mistake of some kind, move aggressively to limit the damage. ***Don't dwell on it!*** Keep following through and you will soon forget about it.

Sometimes we need mistakes. They put us back on track and inform us how we can improve for the next time. A famous philosopher said, *"That which does not kill me only serves to make me stronger!"* Follow through on your efforts; it pays off in the end.

4. Be Responsible. We are all self-employed. It is our job to look after ourselves. You are in charge of the research and development, production, and marketing of the product known as "you." In effect, you own the place known as yourself. You have a responsibility to yourself.

Since you are the primary creative force in your life, you should always look after your best interests. You are the architect of your own destiny, so design a good foundation for yourself. When you finally realize that no one is coming to your rescue, that you are the one who determines everything in your life, you have to go ahead and ***take charge!***

Those who rule must also learn to obey. Obey the orders that you yourself put in motion. If you are dieting for a certain look, follow through by being responsible to yourself and your goal. That means that you should make that special meal even though you don't feel like it. That means that you should do the extra calf work even though you feel tired.

When you set out to do something, you must follow through. Make that commitment to yourself and to your goals. Lock in that goal, and burn your bridges. Don't turn back from your journey. Remember, **you are 100% responsible for what you become.** You own the blueprints to yourself.

If you control yourself through self-discipline, other people can never control you. You call the shots. Whatever you ask of yourself, go ahead and do it with everything you have. You're counting on it. ***Don't let yourself down!*** Be a responsible bodybuilder and run that physique of yours into peak condition.

Those are the psychological principles that will guarantee your success as a bodybuilder. You need that special flame called passion to give you desire; you need goals to direct the flame, and you need self-discipline to keep the fire going. When you put them all together, you'll forge a beautiful body.

THE
ONLY
TIME
YOU'LL FIND
SUCCESS
BEFORE
WORK
IS IN
THE
DICTIONARY.

Chapter 14

The Surprising Truth about Losing Weight After 40

A s you grow older, it often becomes more difficult to manage your weight. However, the reasons may be different than you think. A recent study challenges the conventional wisdom about metabolism across the lifespan.

Rather than slowing down in middle age, human metabolism seems to remain stable from 20 to 60. That's according to a groundbreaking study at Duke University.

That means you could be wasting time and money on expensive supplements and magic foods that claim to help you burn more calories. Try these suggestions, instead, for taking weight off and keeping it off after 40.

Increasing Muscle Mass

While your metabolism may remain strong for decades, your muscle mass starts decreasing sooner. The average adult loses about 3 to 5% every ten years after they turn 30. While some change is inevitable, **slowing the process down can help you stay lean.**

Try these tips:

1. **Use resistance. The key to building strength is contracting your muscles against external resistance.** Experiment with machines, free weights, and body weight exercises to see what works for you.

2. **Train heavy.** For faster results, make your workouts more intense. Use a weight that allows you to just barely complete your last repetition.

3. **Consume adequate protein.** Current guidelines recommend getting 10 to 35% of your calories from protein, and many experts prefer the upper range. Some studies suggest that eating a protein-rich meal or snack within 2 hours after working out is especially helpful.

4. **Schedule rest days.** Your muscles grow while you're recovering in between workouts. You can take it easy or do easier activities like hiking.

Other Tips for Losing Weight After 40

Aging affects your body weight in other ways too. Increases in insulin resistance lead to excess sugar being stored as fat. Hormonal changes play a role too, especially for women after menopause. On top of that, your lifestyle may become more sedentary.

Using these strategies can help:

1. **Choose whole foods.** Satisfy your hunger with natural foods rich in nutrients and fiber and low in added sugar and salt. **Smart choices include vegetables, fruits, whole grains, lean proteins, and healthy fats.**

2. **Drink water.** It's easy to confuse thirst with hunger. Staying hydrated will enhance your digestion and help you feel full.

3. **Limit alcohol.** Many cocktails contain a lot of empty calories, and any alcohol can lower your

resistance to junk food. If you drink, practice moderation.

4. **Sleep well.** Getting 7 to 8 hours of sleep each night is important for your overall wellbeing. Stick to a regular bedtime that allows you to wake up naturally feeling refreshed.

5. **Weigh yourself.** The average adult gains 1 to 2 pounds each year. Using a scale or tape measure at least once a week gives you a chance to make easy corrections before the doughnuts add up.

6. **Move around.** How many hours a day do you spend sitting? **In addition to regular exercise, take a break to stretch and walk around each half hour anytime you're at your desk or watching TV.**

7. **Seek support.** Changing your habits is easier when you have your family and friends on your side. Invite your loved ones to join you in preparing nutritious meals at home and sticking to a workout program.

8. **See your doctor.** If you need more help, talk with your doctor about your personal situation.

For example, a thyroid screening can catch issues that cause weight gain, fatigue, and depression in many adults over 35.

Staying slim after 40 takes a little effort, but the benefits are huge. You lower your risk for many serious health conditions and increase your chances for living a long and active life.

Chapter 15

Who Else Wants a Workout That Reverses Aging?

Y OU PROBABLY KNOW THAT any form of physical activity beats sitting on the couch if you want to look and feel younger. However, **some exercises are more effective than others**. Researchers from the Mayo Clinic figured out how you can design your workouts to reverse the clock as much as possible in as little time as possible.

The Mayo team tested 3 different exercise programs on men and women under 30 and over 65. After 12 weeks, high-intensity interval training (HIIT) proved to be the anti-aging winner, compared to lighter cycling and lifting or strength training alone.

That's because HIIT made changes at the cellular level, enhancing mitochondrial function. Participants over 65 had a 69% increase in their cells' ability to take in oxygen and produce energy, while those under 30 had a 49% boost.

While that might sound a little technical, it means slowing down age-related physical decline, including osteoporosis, arthritis, hypertension, heart conditions, and digestive issues.

Learn how to stay young. Follow these guidelines for a workout program that reverses aging.

High Intensity Interval Training to Fight Aging

1. **Understand the concept. High-intensity interval training means alternating between short periods of intense exercise and gentler activities.** In the Mayo study, this involved 4 minutes of fast cycling followed by 3 minutes of easy cycling repeated 4 times.

2. **Be consistent.** You'll need to do HIIT regularly to see results. Aim for at least 2 to 3 workouts each week.

3. **Proceed gradually.** Avoid injuries by giving your body time to adapt. **You might start out with just a few minutes of HIIT and work your way up slowly to 15 or 20 minutes.**

4. **Rest up.** The gentle periods are just as important as the more intense phase. That's when your body becomes conditioned to return to your normal heart rate quickly.

Strength Training to Fight Aging

1. **Build muscle.** Strength training may not rival HIIT for cellular changes, but it's good at slowing down age-related muscle loss. Otherwise, most adults over 30 lose about 5% each decade.

2. **Challenge yourself. Heavier weights and lower repetitions will give you faster results.** Try picking the biggest dumbbell that you can lift safely 4 to 8 times.

3. **Take time off.** Work hard at the gym, but rest between sessions so muscles can heal and grow. Take a day of rest or do other activities like biking or running.

Other Anti-Aging Training Tips

1. **Steady yourself. Training for balance will protect you from falls and may help prevent**

some forms of dementia. Take a yoga class or practice standing on one foot while you brew coffee.

2. **Stand tall.** Good posture helps you to look younger and puts less strain on your spine. It also enhances bodily functions like respiration, circulation, and digestion.

3. **Target your whole body.** Include lots of full body exercises in your workout. You'll burn more calories and increase your coordination. Plus, you'll see more gains in functional fitness that prepares you to handle real-life tasks like vacuuming and yard work.

4. **Engage your brain.** Your mental health matters too. In addition to exercising your brain with word puzzles, try physical activities that make you think, like waltzing or playing tennis.

5. **Be social.** Connecting with others is like a fountain of youth. Work out with a buddy or go running with your spouse.

Any work out can help you manage your weight and reduce inflammation, but HIIT does more to maintain healthy cell functions as you grow older. Make high intensity interval training part of your formula for fitness and anti-aging.

Chapter 16

Exercises for the Extremely Busy

G ETTING IN A GOOD workout can be challenging, considering how busy most of us are. **A workout doesn't have to involve a lot of equipment or an hour of your time.**

The exercise program that follows is not designed to be a complete program, but it is a worthwhile workout that you can sneak in when you just don't have the time to visit the gym.

If the following exercises are too easy, add weight, more sets, or extra repetitions.

Let's get started:

1. **Pushups.** If you're in great shape, do 100 correctly formed pushups as quickly as possible, taking breaks as needed. If you struggle to do one

good push up, try doing them on your knees, or stand at the base of the stairs and put your hands on the stairs. **The key is to make it easy enough that you can do at least 10-20 repetitions.**

2. **Bodyweight squats.** From a standing position, squat down and stand back up. Do as many as you can and try to go all the way down until your thighs are parallel to the floor. If that's too difficult, grab a doorframe to pull yourself back up.

3. **Jump squats.** These are like the bodyweight squats, but instead of just standing up, you're going to jump as high as you can, land softly, and repeat. Do as many as you can. This is challenging to do.

4. **Lunges.** To lunge, you simply take a big step and then lower yourself down until your back knee just grazes the ground. This one will really help to stretch out your hips and challenge your balance.

5. **Jump lunges.** As you come up from your standard lunge, jump up and switch your legs in the air. Go back down and repeat.

6. **Jump.** Jumping is great exercise. Hop on one foot, jump on two feet, then alternate to hop on the other foot. Use a jump rope if you like. Jump for height or long jump. Jumping is good for your bones and keeps your nervous system sharp.

7. **Stairs.** If you have access to a multi-story building, walk up a few floors and walk back down. If you're in decent shape, try running up the stairs. Who needs a stair machine at the gym?

8. **Planks.** The exercise is so effective because you're harnessing one of your core's most key functions: bracing. Get down on the ground. Stack your elbows directly beneath your shoulders and extend your legs. Rest your weight on your elbows and your toes. Squeeze your glutes and core to create full-body tension. Think about pulling your belly button into your spine Contract your low back, lats, and rhomboids. Your back should form a straight line; don't let your pelvis dip down or your butt to rise. Face your gaze face down, which keeps your neck in a neutral position. It's better to hold a truly focused plank for 30 seconds to a minute than to hold a lousy plank for 4 consecutive minutes.

Getting a good workout can be as simple using your body for resistance. **These exercises don't require a lot of room or any fancy equipment.** Just the pushups, bodyweight squats, and planks are enough to keep most folks in decent shape.

These exercises can be just as challenging as they are beneficial to you. The key is to perform them with proper form, so don't be afraid to ask for help regarding how to perform these exercises correctly. In fact, if you have any questions regarding these movements, feel free to contact me at (318) 550-0050. I'm more than happy to help keeping you safe while getting the results you're wanting.

Give these exercises a try the next time you're short on time. You'll be pleased with the results.

Chapter 17

The Psychology Of Peak Condition

FOR THE PURPOSE OF THIS CONTENT, WE CONSIDER EVERY INDIVIDUAL, MALE OR FEMALE, THAT IS TRYING TO TRANSFORM THEIR PHYSIQUE A BODYBUILDER.

I like your attitude. The fact that you are reading this book sets you apart from millions of other people, both physically and mentally. By choosing fitness as your lifestyle, you've made a deliberate choice to improve yourself. That makes you a doer and not a watcher.

If you are truly ready to begin dieting, I must tell you something very important: *you are going to war!* A psychological war. It will be against your toughest opponent - *yourself!*

It is a war that has littered the field of physical culture with many casualties. You could receive serious injuries to your self-esteem. Or you might have your self-discipline shot apart. You may even have your enthusiasm killed.

Once you start to diet, you'll encounter all kinds of traps, traitors, and temptations along the way. Only a handful of dieters will remain unscathed. Those who make it through will be heavily rewarded. They will be called heroes.

In truth, it is simple to become sliced. Armed with the advice in this book, you can take your physique to the exact condition you want, and I do mean exact. However, I didn't say it was easy. As a matter of fact, it's very tough. Many bodybuilders lose the battle. And the toughest part of the battle - the one that determines whether you win or lose - **occurs right in your mind.**

At a state competition, three bodybuilders from various weight classes dropped out before the show. One of them did so because he feared a certain competitor would be there. Another one bailed out because he was burned out from training. (He had only two weeks left to go.) The third person had blown her diet, largely because of personal problems.

After an entire year of strict dieting, gut-wrenching workouts, and huge personal sacrifices, they defeated themselves before they even got to the contest site. These are psychological casualties.

Of those who did grace the stage, many showed up way off their mark. No doubt head games were responsible for this as well. And while the faces and places may change, and so may the level of competition, the story remains the same.

All of these individuals could have avoided their disappointments.

That's the main purpose of this chapter.

I don't want to lose a single person to the battle of physical excellence. You should reach your intended physical condition every time out of the chute.

And you will! I will take you down the hallways of your mind and show you where the enemy hides out. The covert operations of the enemy will be fully exposed for you to see. Once you know their plan of attack, you can maneuver your mind accordingly to smash their offensive. This way, you will always know which direction you're going.

A well-known psychologist once said it best: "If you don't know where you want to go, you will probably end up somewhere else." Carefully apply what this chapter offers, and success will be yours.

The Power of Passion

During a seminar Arnold Schwarzenegger was giving, a skinny teenage boy stood up and asked, "Arnold, I want to become a professional bodybuilder. What must I know to make it happen?"

Arnold looked at the boy with a knowing glance and said, "Unless you go to bed with a burning desire to turn pro, and wake up with a burning desire to turn pro, you might as well forget it, because that determines everything!"

The boy replied, "What if I don't feel that way?"

Arnold responded, "Well, you look kind of tall. Maybe you should play basketball!"

As complex as human behavior may seem, when you are dealing with a desire to get cut, you are actually dealing with an emotion. ***Somewhere in your past, something happened to you to give you a powerful urge to change your body.*** Whatever did happen, the logical part of your brain joins in and starts supplying you with reasons you should continue that urge. The more moving the experience was, or the higher the degree of arousal at the time it occurred, the stronger the emotion and also the rationalization behind the drive. When the motion becomes intense, ***it turns into a passion.***

Once passion is put into action, you become unstoppable. It makes you relentless. When this emotion takes over, a huge reservoir of mental and physical energy comes pouring into your life. Suddenly your body needs less sleep. Any barrier that lies in your path seems to be a minor inconvenience. Passion is the driving force behind the movers and the shakers in this world.

Arnold's numerous bodybuilding and acting successes are because of passion. Frank Sinatra singing into his 70s, and George Burns doing films in his eighties. You see, it doesn't matter what area of life you're in, if you love what you are doing, you keep forging ahead.

Clearly, it's passion that fuels the famous.

You need this emotion. Passion makes you train harder, prevents you from cheating, and gives you energy when scientific knowledge says you shouldn't have any. Of course, you can get into shape without this powerful emotion, but it will become very difficult and wearisome. With passion, you turn into a fighter! Your efforts carry much more oomph behind them. Remember, *superior rewards go to superior efforts.*

Don't worry if you currently lack passion. You may have entered bodybuilding ever so quietly and casually, and never had a significant emotional experience to spark your interest. That's fine. The following list of points is designed to increase the enthusiasm behind your drive:

Never consider failure. Once you make a decision, put everything you have into it. Do not think for a moment that you will fall short of your desires. Otherwise, fear will creep in and weaken your passion severely. **Fear is the greatest enemy of human potential.** On the other hand, the individual filled with passion is a fearless competitor. That person believes in all of his or her actions and consequently progresses faster than people of little faith. Fix your thoughts on success.

Seize every moment. At every given moment, try to do the most productive thing possible to improve your transformation journey. When you analyze the dieting methods of successful and unsuccessful bodybuilder, you find they basically use the same procedures to get prepared for a contest. **The difference in their physiques comes from the fact the winners do more every moment**

while they are dieting. They weigh all foods, keep accurate calorie counts, check their bodies more often under various lighting conditions, and so forth. **Make every moment count, and you'll be amazed at your progress. Your passion will grow as a result.**

Forget the past. Live in the here and now. It does not matter whether your upbringing was ideal or unpleasant. You are the master of your destiny, and the present is all you have to act on. Few things are more depressing than listening to a person tell you how he "used to look" or what might have really happened to his/her physique had he/she known back then what is known now. Give me a break. Every individual who whines about the past is full of apathy. His passion left him when gas was 32 cents a gallon. There will never be a better time than now, so give it everything you have - today.

Speak the language of winners. Never start off any of your sentences with these phrases: *"I can't," "We'll see," "I'll try," "If only I had...,"* *""I'd better not," "It probably won't,"* or *"I never will."* I could list more confidence-destroying statement, but these make the point. Simply put, when our self-instructions are negative, our actions will also be negative. We can only do what our programs tell us to do. Therefore, speak like a winner.

You'd be amazed how often winners answer a question with a resounding yes, while losers give all kinds of vague and wishy-washy affirmatives or excuses. Excuses are for losers! Think about it for a second. Does the winner have to make excuses for his success? No! It's always the losers who make excuses for why they didn't win. Remember this fact!

Avoid negative people. Their constant barrage of gloom and doom carries a message into your subconscious. Of course, it doesn't happen overnight; the process is slow and insidious. But don't underestimate its effect on your emotions. And don't think of trying to convert such a person into your line of thought. You see, negative people don't know they're negative. They think they're being realistic and everyone else is screwed up!

Believe in yourself. Set no limits whatsoever on your potential. Forget the notion that you can only bench press or squat so much weight. Without even knowing you, I know that you haven't even begun to tap into your potential. That's not hype, it's the truth!

Fill your mind with the belief that your physique is far more amazing than you now believe it to be. Remember, when it comes to bodybuilding, your major barriers are your own self-limitations.

If you totally expect to bring up a lagging body part, everything aligns itself consciously and subconsciously to make that desire come true. The more you believe in yourself, the more passion you attach to all of your actions.

Develop a sense of urgency. When people are full of passion, they can't wait to get things done. You can spot such people easily. They have a purpose in their walk, a certain look in their eyes, and you notice them as soon as they enter a room. You can develop this kind of essence yourself.

The Greatness of Goals

Before you spend the next several months dieting, you should spend a few minutes defining what you want. You'd be surprised how many bodybuilders have vaguely defined goals. Sure, they'd like to get more cut, or get bigger, but that's not concrete enough. These desires are far too general. **You need to get specific.** The mind loves to focus on all kinds of little details. How much bigger do you need to be?

Start out by breaking down your ultimate goal and setting for yourself some short-term, easily obtainable goals. You should decide to lose four pounds in two weeks, or one inch off your waistline in 20 days. The more precise you are, the better. Taken over a period of time, these little goals have a big way of adding up to dramatic results. Goals give your workouts a sense of meaning and purpose. **The more you know what you want, and the more effort you put into it, the more clearly defined will be the result.**

This is a very powerful concept, and it must not be taken lightly. Goals are extremely important for success. They direct all of that passion.

To help you in your physique transformation progress, here are a few points you should know about goals:

1. Burn Goals into Your Subconscious. When you write down goals, they become easier to stick to and harder to neglect. Besides, writing down your goals brings to your attention what should be done.

2. Make Goals Realistic. Whenever you choose a goal, make sure it's totally believable to you. Keep in mind that it doesn't matter who else believes in your goals. Take my advice, don't even bother to tell others. It's totally unimportant for your success. You are the one behind the driver's wheel, and they aren't even in your backseat!

The key point is this: when the goal is realistic and believable to you, it will happen. If you don't really believe it can be done, but you're hoping it might, it will never happen. There are no gray areas at all.

3. *Update Goals Constantly.* It's amazing how many folks drift away from their goal-setting techniques once they gain some good results. And yet, real bodybuilding is an ongoing process. **The key word in bodybuilding is *building*.** Look at how many people continue to improve year after year, while others look absolutely identical year after year.

Of course, the ones who don't improve have all the answers. They blame it on genetics, or on the fact that they haven't used some exotic drug. Nothing could be further from the truth.

Successful people keep improving simply because they refuse to be satisfied with attaining just one goal. They constantly create new goals. They see something that they want, and they think, "I want that, too!" Bingo, they have just updated their goal. Then they go ahead and make the necessary changes in their diet and training, and pretty soon they get what they are looking for. ***That is the real secret to physique transformation success!***

4. Do It Now. Strange as it may seem, many bodybuilders know exactly what their physique needs, but they won't go ahead and get it. They are putting it off until they are ready. To them, doing it right now is too soon. Everything has to be perfect, and then they will go ahead. "What needs to be perfect," you may ask. There are thousands of different excuses, and none of them hold water. Remember, ***excuses are for losers!***

Someone who wants to procrastinate can think of any excuse. And when a person does it often enough, the rationalization for the delay simply becomes an everyday excuse. Truth is, there is always some form of inconvenience or stress in everyday life. Superior people function despite this. The more time you waste making excuses, the more you delay your reward. It's already rightfully yours; you just have to invest the time in order to take it.

The main reason some people don't invest the time is that they fear the work. To them, it's too much effort to change the way things are. They have encountered the Comfort Zone! Simply put, this is a place where people have grown so comfortable and complacent that they do not wish to alter their lives greatly, when doing so would markedly increase their progress. **Make no mistake about it, the Comfort Zone is a deep rut!** And pardon me for being blunt, but the only difference between being in a rut and being in a grave is death!

The Comfort Zone has ruined many of people who have great potential. It kind of sneaks up on you until all of your efforts are feeble ones at best. Then you become one of the dreaded "nothings." The worst part of the Comfort Zone is that people do it to themselves. Yet, they will never accept responsibility for their own lack of effort.

Excuses, excuses. This person simply doesn't want to make the necessary changes in his diet or training. That's because these changes would mean a greater effort on his part. The truth is that this person has the chance to make the move, and he's not acting on it.

There really is nothing holding you back, because there's nothing to fear. Dealing with fear is really very simple. Move away from what you fear, and pretty soon it will dominate your life. Move toward your fear, and it gets smaller. That's the difference between cowardice and courage. Become full of courage! Start those goals now.

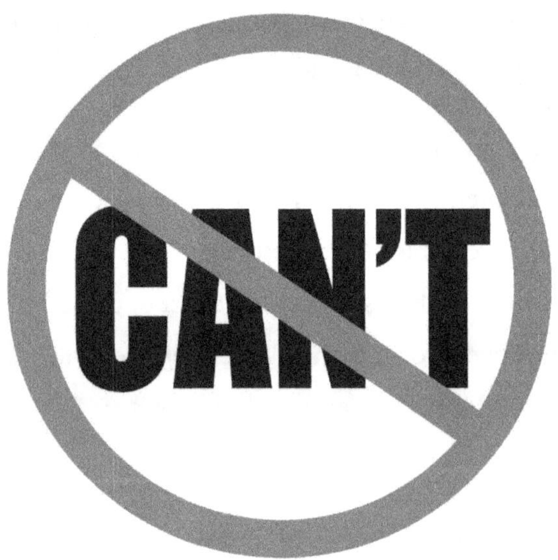

ELIMINATE THIS WORD!

Stop thinking you can't do things and start thinking you can. It's important to eliminate negatives from your vocabulary, especially the word "can't." When you begin to think positively , you'll find yourself attempting and succeeding at more things. Remember, by eliminating the negatives you'll let the positives come through.

Chapter 18

7 Benefits of Strength Training Besides Building Muscle

L IFTING WEIGHTS IS THE natural choice if you want a broad back and bulging biceps. However, you might be surprised to learn that it's also effective for a much wider range of fitness goals.

Less than 25% of American adults exercise regularly. Even fewer make strength training a central part of their routine. If that sounds like you, you're missing out on more than bigger muscles.

Incorporating the power of resistance into your workouts can help you get more impressive results in less time.

Learn more about what strength training can do for you, and how to get started.

7 Lesser-Known Benefits of Strength Training:

1. **Condition your heart.** Aerobics may be the first thing that comes to mind when you think about exercises for your heart, but strength training works, too. That's because it helps reduce abdominal fat that causes inflammation and other health issues.

2. **Lower your blood pressure.** Hypertension puts you at higher risk for stroke and heart disease, and there are often no symptoms to warn you. Along with taking any medication recommended by your doctor, physical activity can help you stay within a safer range.

3. **Lose weight.** Muscle burns more calories than fat even when you're sitting on the couch. As long as you avoid eating more, you may find it easier to shed excess pounds.

4. **Prevent falls.** Enhancing your balance and posture makes you steadier on your feet. Weight-bearing exercises also thicken your bones, so your injuries may be less serious even if you do slip.

5. **Increase flexibility.** Lowering weights affects

your body in much the same way as static stretches. That extra flexibility reduces stress and gives you greater freedom of movement.

6. **Increase your energy.** Daily tasks require less effort when you reduce your body fat and learn to use your body more efficiently. You may find it easier to keep up with your children and grandchildren.

7. **Boost your overall wellbeing.** Research shows that exercise can be as effective as antidepressants for some patients. In addition to looking fit, you're likely to feel happier and calmer and may even reverse cognitive decline associated with aging.

Tips for Getting Started with Strength Training:

1. **Follow instructions.** Lifting weights can be safe as long as you take a few simple precautions. Work with a trainer or watch videos to study proper form and choose exercises that are less likely to cause injury.

2. **Proceed gradually.** Start with light weights and work your way up as your body adapts. As a general rule, expect to increase your load by 10% or less at any single time.

3. **Lift heavy.** At the same time, you'll progress faster if you use the heaviest weights you can handle safely. That usually means you can just barely complete your last repetition.

4. **Seek variety.** Work your muscles from different angles. Experiment with free weights and machines and body weight exercises, like pushups and dips.

5. **Take days off.** Your muscles actually grow during the time you spend resting in between workouts. That might mean relaxing or doing other activities like hiking or swimming.

6. **Adjust your lifestyle.** Adopt healthy habits to go along with your physical activities. Eat a balanced diet and aim for 8 hours of sleep each night. Manage stress and cultivate mutually supportive relationships.

A toned body looks great, but strength training offers so much more. Take care of your body and mind with a well-rounded fitness program that will help you enjoy a long and active life.

Chapter 19

Body Transformation Secrets

What You Can Learn From Bodybuilders

B ODYBUILDERS ARE COMMONLY THE butt of jokes, but anyone that is trying to change the appearance of their body could learn a lot from bodybuilders.

Did you know that the current diets recommended for weight loss by physicians are the same diets that bodybuilders have been using for years?

Bodybuilders are always current. They're constantly on the lookout for new information that can give them an edge. Many of them search the latest research publications looking for information about fat loss and muscle gain.

Plus, bodybuilders are the best at transforming their bodies.

Consider the following ideas you could learn from a bodybuilder:

1. You probably need more protein. While it's true that you don't need a lot of protein to sustain life, your body composition will improve if your protein intake increases, within a reasonable limit.

- Protein is also metabolically expensive. **It takes a lot of energy for your body to digest and process protein.** It's not easy to convert protein into carbohydrates for fuel or into fat for storage.

2. Strength training is one of the best aerobic activities. If you move quickly between exercises and minimize the rest periods between sets, **there is nothing short of sprinting that will get your heart beating faster.** This also requires that you do the proper exercises. For example, squatting instead of performing leg curls.

3. Strength training is the best calorie burning activity. Many other activities burn more calories during the exercise period itself. However, the calorie burning stops when you stop performing those other activities.

- The muscle damage caused by lifting weights takes days to repair. **Your metabolism is increased during that entire period.**

4. Carbohydrates are a significant issue. Most natural bodybuilders keep their protein and fat intakes quite constant, regardless of their goals. The only macronutrient they manipulate is the carbohydrates.

- When they want to gain weight, the carbohydrates increase. When it's time to lose weight, they decrease their carbohydrate intake.

5. They always keep up with their cardio. Cardio training is used by bodybuilders to stay healthy and lean, recover from muscle building workouts, and to keep calories higher during dieting periods. A little bit of cardiovascular exercise is always a good idea.

- **However, they also don't do a lot of cardio.** Weight loss is primarily a function of their diet.

6. Bodybuilders are maniacal when it comes to tracking workouts and food intake. While the average person doesn't need to know exactly how many calories they ate, most people couldn't even guess how many they ate today. What adjustments will you make if your results are sub-par? You can't make any if you don't know your food intake.

- Do you know what the same workout, over and

over, gets you? The same body you already have. Bodybuilders are always recording their workouts and increasing either the weight or the number of repetitions with each workout.

- When they fail to progress, they change the workout.

7. Bodybuilders track progress. Any intelligent bodybuilder regularly weighs himself, records regular body-part measurements, and takes full-body pictures. They change their diet or exercise routine often. **When do YOU change your diet and workout?**

8. They are consistent and patient. When a bodybuilder is dieting, he might be trying to only lose half a pound a week. His goal might be to only gain 1 pound per month during weight gain phases. They essentially never miss a workout or their daily caloric goals.

The average person doesn't require the same level of commitment as a bodybuilder, but there are many things you could do if you want to transform your body. Take a few tips from bodybuilders and your time spent in the gym and kitchen will be much more productive.

Chapter 20

Why I Love Bodybuilding

And Yes! You're A Bodybuilder!

A T ONE POINT OR another, most of us all have dreamed of greatness. For some, that means becoming a lawyer or a doctor. For others, it's success in the movie industry, and a few dreams of becoming a professional athlete. I have the utmost respect for people who dare to dream the impossible dream, for only those that seek to achieve greatness ever have a chance of rising above mediocrity. My dream had always been to become a successful doctor, fitness professional... and yes, a bodybuilder.

However, to me, bodybuilding is not just stepping on stage in a pair of trunks and posing for 90 seconds. I know most outsiders really break down the sport to that one simple act. But, bodybuilding is so much more.

To me, bodybuilding (or Physique Transformation as I prefer to call it) is the 43-year-old guy who goes

from a fat, bloated 240 pounds to a muscular 201. It's the 18-year-old kid who sets a goal to squat 315 pounds and achieves it. It's the half-crazed woman getting ready for her first fitness contest. And it's the 45-year-old mom just wanting to look better and have more energy. To really understand the sport of bodybuilding, you have to look at the overall picture. It's not only what you see in the magazines. How many of you really compete? Although most of you don't, I'm sure you all consider yourselves bodybuilders.

I've met some of the greatest people in the world in the gym. Occasionally, I'm lucky enough to work with some of them. I recently worked with a very successful business executive. Here was a guy who makes tons of money, yet he was literally killing himself every day because of his sedentary lifestyle. Sure, he was rich, but when you're 45 and heading for a heart attack at 50, what's the point? He made the decision to get off his butt and into the gym. When I met him, he was a portly 310 pounds. At the time of our last session together, he was down to a muscular 245 and he had dropped quite a few pant sizes along the way. That's a physique transformation! ***That's what bodybuilding is!***

I get countless questions each day about exercise and diet. Some of them I answer, some of them I don't. If I feel I can help someone help themselves, I'll usually do the best I can to help them improve themselves. So many people consider bodybuilding an individual sport, but it really isn't. Think about how many people have helped you along the way to achieving your personal physique transformation goals. The guy in the gym who came over to help with your form or your friends that pushed you to keep going to the gym. Certainly, no one can force you to go to the gym; no one can force you to eat 6 meals a day. Those are all things that are ultimately up to you. However, I know from personal experience that part of the reason why I'm able to do these things is from the motivation I get from others.

Recently I've been training several women. Obviously, I'm not dealing with females that have aspirations of being the next Ms. Olympia. However, the dedication that these ladies exhibit is remarkable. I have these women doing exercises that other people look at and just shake their heads. In a very short time period, one of these ladies has dropped 24 pounds of body fat. Certainly, she could not have done it without my help, but neither could I have helped her accomplish her goals without her drive and dedication. I can see daily changes in this woman's physique and overall attitude. The motivation that gives me is unbelievable. ***That's what bodybuilding is all about!***

The camaraderie in the sport is something I've never experienced anywhere else. As a kid, I experienced the close-knit bond of competitive swimming at an extremely high level. Very few people get to share in something that special. Through my participation in bodybuilding, I've been lucky enough to feel like I'm part of something special again. Maybe it's the fact that we are so different from the rest of society that brings bodybuilders so closely together. Sure, there's more than enough backstabbing and infighting within the sport. However, there's also a shared feeling of being part of something special. Until you have felt that burn from a brutal workout, or until you've spent time gritting your teeth on rep after rep, it's not possible to understand what I'm talking about.

So, what is bodybuilding?

Bodybuilding is the quest to develop yourself into ***your own idea of perfection.*** For some, that's developing a physique that will turn heads at the beach. For others, it's achieving a level of development that will win a bodybuilding contest. **For most, it's simply something people do to stay healthy and look fit.**

Whatever your goals, no other sport will transform your body like bodybuilding. **It's fascinating to see how fast someone can completely change their physique through proper training and nutrition.** Seeing the fruits of your labor in the mirror is like an extremely addictive motivator. The more results you see, the further you want to improve. To me, that's what bodybuilding is all about.

OK. I know I'm going to take some heat for this one. If you haven't seen Bill Phillips' "Body For Life" video tape, the one he produced in 1998, I really recommend that you try to get a copy. When I first received the tape in the mail, I had a terrible attitude about it. *"Christ, here we go again, another shameless plug for EAS supplements."* **I was wrong and I have to be honest with you.** I found this to be the most inspirational bodybuilding video I have seen. Sure, I've seen many of the Mr. Olympia tapes and other tapes by pro bodybuilders. Certainly, watching these behemoths train is inspirational and awe-inspiring. But, that's all they are - videos of pros working out. As bodybuilders, we all face daily challenges in our lives that sometimes make it difficult to eat, train, or retain a positive focus on our bodybuilding goals. "The Body For Life" tape details the story of 10 people, some who had to overcome some pretty tough obstacles, who made amazing physique transformations. No. It's not a hard-core training tape. It's a bodybuilding tape, showing you people much like yourself ***achieving their idea of the perfect physique.*** I probably watched this tape twice a month until I foolishly misplaced it. And it inspired me every time I watched it!

Bodybuilding certainly isn't a sport for everybody. Most people lack the necessary drive and discipline that's required to be successful at any level. For the few of us who do, it's a fantastic feeling. It's hard for me to convey how much I truly enjoy the sport, but it's definitely a wonderful journey. Bodybuilding has given me the opportunity to help a lot of people, and it has allowed me to share in the feeling of victory when one of these people proudly speaks of achieving their goals with a sparkle in their eyes. There's not a better feeling in the world. Nothing makes me more complete than knowing I helped someone take control of their life. When you're a bodybuilder, it's easy to get wrapped up in yourself and your own dreams and aspirations. I think many of you will find that the best motivator is sometimes helping someone else achieve their goals. That's what this book is about. To me, that's what bodybuilding is all about.

BODY TRANSFORMATION

is not a matter of having good genetics,

but making the most of the genetics you have.

Chapter 21

What to do now...

Here's How To Get Started On That Healthy And Fit Body You Have Always Dreamed Of

IF YOU HAVE ARRIVED on this page after reading this entire book, then thank you and congratulations. I can't wait for you to implement the strategies in **Small Steps Every Day**.

Now this is where the average person stops. The average person reads a book, gets inspired, but ultimately takes no action.

Simply by making it to the very end of this book tells me you're not average. You're a person who is motivated to improve your quality of life, and I'm passionate about helping you do that.

I hope you now feel motivated to take action and start transforming yourself into the person you envision being using **Small Steps Every Day**.

As you now know, by implementing the strategies outlined in this book, you're can achieve a much higher-quality life, while having plenty of time to live your life to the fullest, not just endure it.

That being said, the next step for you is simple:

Get started!

Taking action is your immediate step. Nothing happens until you make it happen. You now have everything you need to add health and fitness into your life.

Still not sure of where to start, or exactly what to do?

I'm more than happy to help you get everything in place, and getting you that health and fit body.

If you'd like me to help, reach out to me by calling me at (318) 550-0050. If you enjoyed this book, you'll do even better with me leading the way.

I'm good at what I do, just like you're good at what you do.

Instead of trying to figure everything out yourself, let me help you dial in your new health and nutrition program. I help folks just like you find the time to add health and fitness into their busy lives. And stick to it.

Here's exactly how we'll do it together:

Step 1: We'll spend time together outlining and developing your training program, nutrition, and overall strategy to fully dial in the perfect solution for you and the time you have.

Step 2: We'll begin integrating your training and nutrition habits into your busy schedule.

Step 3: We'll dial everything in from your training to your nutrition to make adding healthy habits into your busy life a walk in the park.

Step 4: Once we have your habits down pat, we will monitor everything to guarantee everything is working seamlessly to get you the greatest results in the shortest time.

Most people think it takes years of hard work and countless hours of working out and preparing meals in advance to get or stay healthy and fit.

Truth is, my done-with-you program is designed to make it an easy and stress-free transition for you, so we give you everything you need to ensure your success in the shortest possible time.

If you're ready to add optimal health into your life and gets twice the results in half the time, let's get on the phone for a no-obligation call with me by going to (318) 550-0050.

Okay, it's time to close this book and take action to make it happen.

I look forward to hearing from you, and more importantly, working together to transform your health and fitness to a much more rewarding level than it is today.

As I said earlier, that's what I do every day and I enjoy helping people like you become the best version of yourself.

To your continued success and enjoying the life you deserve to live.

Jack Ward. M.D.

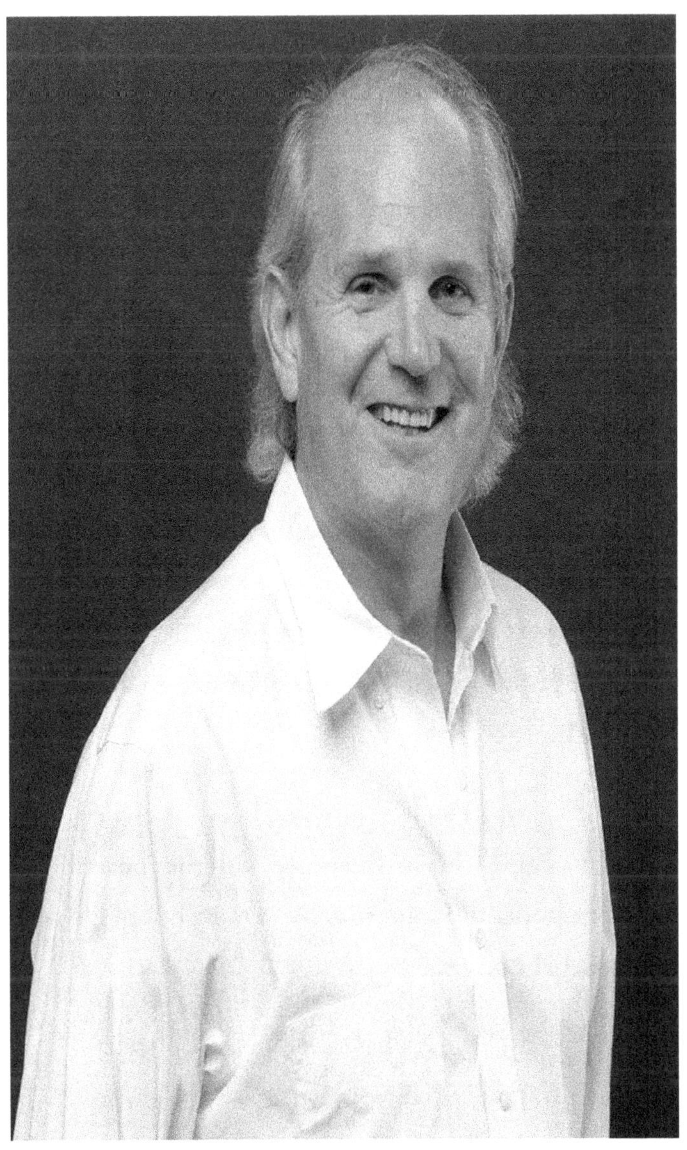

About The Author

Who Is Dr. Jack Ward?

Dr. Jack is an innovator in optimal health and longevity. For over four decades, he has been a respected member of the healthcare industry. He has established himself as a leader in promoting alternatives to the conventional medical model of sick care. He has a keen understanding of how to personalize medical care for each client. This patient-focus approach has earned him a special place in the healthcare community.

Dr. Jack's patients include athletes, business owners, and everyday people who are frustrated with the conventional sick-care model and want to achieve more out of life with **Purposeful Longevity**.

Along the way, Dr. Jack has developed proprietary protocols to build effective longevity and to ensure people have their best health. His program, **Purposeful**

Longevity, helps people match an optimal healthspan to their lifespan.

Dr. Jack enjoys his professional life, but it takes a back seat to spending valuable time with his spouse and friends. His priority is to build a medical practice around his life, not his life around business.

Dr. Jack is a physician-leader in heart health and longevity. He has over 40 years of experience with patient care since receiving his medical degree from the Louisiana State University School of Medicine. For the past twenty years, his focus has been on optimal health through nutrition and exercise, heart health, and longevity. He continues to study innovative approaches in medicine to include in his crusade for helping his clients/patients achieving **Purposeful Longevity**.